In My Hands

In My Hands

My Parents' Journey to the Other Side

Barbara Lorello

Strategic Book Publishing and Rights Co.

Copyright © 2020 Barbara Lorello. All rights reserved.

No part of this book may be reproduced or transmitted in any form or by any means, graphic, electronic, or mechanical, including photocopying, recording, taping, or by any information storage retrieval system, without the permission, in writing, of the publisher. For more information, email support@sbpra.net, Attention: Subsidiary Rights.

Strategic Book Publishing & Rights Co., LLC
USA | Singapore
www.sbpra.net

For information about special discounts for bulk purchases, please contact Strategic Book Publishing and Rights Co. Special Sales, at bookorder@sbpra.net.

ISBN: 978-1-951530-22-8

Dedication

To Mom and Dad: I am grateful for the opportunity to give in a way none of us imagined.

To my beloved Geno: Thank you for loving me and my parents and thank you for helping me let them die with dignity. I couldn't have done it without you.

And to my sons, Joe and Alex: Thank you for seeing me for who I really am, not how others wanted you to see me.

Table of Contents

Introduction	ix
Preface	xi
Chapter One – The Beginning	1
Chapter Two – The Fall	6
Chapter Three – Thanksgiving	9
Chapter Four – The Medical System	13
Chapter Five – The Hospice Angels	39
Chapter Six – The Wedding	59
Chapter Seven – The Unexpected	66
Chapter Eight – The First Ending	68
Chapter Nine – A New Beginning	85
Chapter Ten – A Turn for the Worse	96
Chapter Eleven – Our Overnight Angel	100
Chapter Twelve – A Second Ending	103
Chapter Thirteen – Funeral Preparations	110
Chapter Fourteen – The Practical Piece	114
Chapter Fifteen – The Spiritual Piece (or Peace)	124
Chapter Sixteen – The Relationship Effect	128
Chapter Seventeen – Pay it Forward	130
Chapter Eighteen – Closure	132

Introduction

In 2009, I relocated to Connecticut to be closer to my parents in their golden years. I wanted to spend time with them and not live life regretting that I hadn't. I never expected that would turn into them literally putting their lives in my hands. These pages will bring you through my journey of the illnesses of both my parents and the challenges we faced.

I hope I can offer some practical and spiritual advice that will help you, or someone you love, in allowing a person to die with dignity. This journey is not for the faint of heart or someone who craves drama. Helping someone die is for those who are steeped in faith and love, and those who have a strong sense of service to others.

Preface

In 2005, I divorced after a twenty-year marriage to a man that was the father to my two sons. It was a challenging time, and the divorce was nasty, to say the least. Two innocent people, my sons, were the ones that were hurt the worst, as my now ex-husband manipulated their view of me with lies about money, supposed affairs, and his version of deceit.

During this time, my sons were extremely confused and wanted to believe everything that their father told them about me. Hence, we became estranged, and I forced communication during this time because I didn't want to lose contact with them. They were my everything, and my ex knew it.

I spent months impatiently waiting for them to see the light. I knew that eventually they would know everything their father was telling them were lies—that I never cheated on him, stole money from him, or lied to him about anything.

I was living in North Carolina at the time, and both of my sons had followed their father to live in Florida. I was happy for them; after all, I lived in Florida in my early twenties, and it was a blast—warm weather, sandy beaches, and plenty of entertainment, but the other side was that I missed them, and I was alone. Not to say that I didn't have friends, but family was some seven hundred miles away, which prevented me from stopping in for Sunday dinner, or most other occasions for that matter.

I had always kept in close contact with my parents in Connecticut, who still lived in the house I grew up in. It was in early 2007 when I started to make changes in my life that would allow me to move closer them. At the time they were in their early seventies, still healthy, but had little to no support as they continued to age. Since my brother lived in Florida and was raising his children, and my sister was living in New Jersey with her own set of personal problems, I was the obvious choice to make the move. Not that I even consulted them, my siblings that is.

I shifted my career to make it more feasible to transfer from North Carolina to Connecticut. I had been in management my whole life, so I began a career at a large retail company that had stores throughout the United States. I also listed my house for sale.

It took a couple of years for everything to align, but in 2009 I loaded my three cats into a cargo van and made the 760-mile trek to a new life in Connecticut.

When I finally settled in Connecticut and got my rhythm at a new job, I spent my time off from work with my parents. I went to their home and cooked, played cards, and laughed with them. Oh, how we laughed! Those were the times I had envisioned when I was living in North Carolina. They were easy, funny, and memorable.

Fast forward to 2015 when things changed. Old age and years of a harried life began to take its toll on my mother and father.

Chapter One

The Beginning

In 1991, on my youngest son's first birthday, my father was diagnosed with an esophageal tumor, a very aggressive cancer. After undergoing a lengthy surgery to remove the tumor that had tripled in size in a matter of weeks, the doctors only gave my father six months to live.

That was the beginning of a spiritual journey that led me to my strong faith in God and his power to make miracles happen. I recall entering the church I had attended during my childhood and making a deal with God. I told him that I wasn't ready to let my father go yet, and that if he would help him live, I would give up smoking (the very thing that caused my father's cancer). I kept my end of the bargain, and so did he.

It was also the time that I entered therapy. During my father's recuperation, chemo, and radiation treatments, my mother dove into a deep depression, which landed her in the psych ward of a local hospital. My father's cancer was something she couldn't control, which sent her off the deep end. When her best friend had her admitted to the hospital for treatment, it left me feeling out of control.

At the time, I was in my late twenties, had two children in diapers, and lived in Florida, which could have been in a different galaxy. I felt helpless to aid my parents. I couldn't take my father for treatments, nor could my mother, and I couldn't help her get out of bed each day. I was completely at a loss.

I don't recall how much time went by, but within days I began to reach out to look for help. It was during my therapy that I learned that both of my parents had struggled throughout their lives with mental illness. My mother, although never formally diagnosed, was somewhat manic, with a sprinkling of bipolar disease, and my father was much the same.

Being raised by these parents left me with little coping skills. I was an insecure, subservient person who hated it when people got mad. It was during that time that I met an amazing psychologist who helped me learn what I needed to live life fully and with some semblance of normalcy. It took six years of weekly sessions to learn how to raise my own children in a healthy environment and live with a man who had his own set of issues.

My parents' mental illness came with its own set of circumstances. One area of concern I always had was their physical health. Both of my parents had what I call "white coat syndrome." For years they went to the doctor on a regular basis and always walked out with another slip of paper for some medication to combat whatever new symptom they had discussed with him. What was more alarming is the things they didn't discuss. It was as if they felt that illness didn't exist if they didn't talk about it.

For years they only talked about the medical issues they wanted to, and for the most part, they were treated for only those illnesses that showed up on blood tests or through some instrument like a blood pressure cuff.

***

Prior to moving back to Connecticut, after my divorce, I dated here and there. I dabbled in Internet dating, went out with some locals, but wasn't really into that scene. During this time, my sons were living in Florida. I had very little communication with them, which was their choice. I missed my kids. A friend recommended that I join Facebook so that I could keep tabs on the kids, since we weren't speaking on a regular basis, so I did. I reconnected with a bunch of friends I hadn't heard from in years. It was fun to catch up with people and see where life had taken them. One of the friends I reconnected with was a guy that my sister had dated in her teens. I remembered him as tall and geeky but someone who was just a nice guy. He and I spent many hours chatting online about where life had taken us since we were teenagers.

He had married someone from his high school, had two daughters and a colorful career. He too was divorced after years of an unhappy marriage. I told him of my plans to move north after I sold my house, and that I had a feeling we would be good friends. We just hit it off.

In early spring of 2008, I got a call from my mother while I was at work. She sounded like hell. She told me she had the flu and that my father was being transported to the hospital after having a heart attack. I was seven hundred miles away.

Through my conversations with Gene, my newfound friend from years gone by, I learned that he lived in Middletown, literally a block from the hospital my father was being transported to. With my mother ill and my sister over three hours away in New Jersey, there was no one close enough to help. So, fast thinking made me call Gene.

"I know this is a lot to ask, but my dad is having a heart attack and is being transported to Middlesex Hospital. I'm on my way up, but it will take me twelve hours to get there. Is there any chance you could go over to the hospital and check on him? My mom has the flu, so she can't."

I had also learned through chatting with Gene that he had stayed in touch with my parents throughout the years. They exchanged Christmas cards and he occasionally visited them, so he had no problem with my request to check in on my dad.

After he visited my dad, he called me with an update. "He's stable and resting," Gene reassured me. "I'll check on him later today and let you know how he is."

I thanked him profusely and felt a huge sense of relief as I continued to drive.

When I finally arrived in Connecticut, I phoned Gene to let him know I got there safely. My travel the night before was treacherous, as a heavy storm dumped so much snow on the highway that I had to stop driving and hunker down for the night. During that phone call, I suggested that Gene and I get together for dinner.

"We can catch up, and you can consider it my way of saying thank you for checking in on my dad." So, we planned to meet for a simple dinner the very next day.

When I tell you that the meeting was surreal, that is an understatement. We reconnected in the lobby of the hotel where I had decided to stay for the night. When I saw Gene for the first time in thirty years, he was slightly grayer and a little heavier than I remembered, but he had blossomed from the geeky guy with big glasses and even bigger hair into a distinguished-looking man in his late forties.

During dinner, we caught up on thirty years. He recounted his twenty-year marriage to a woman he never loved, the birth of both of his daughters (I could tell instantly that they were the light in his life), his career in college athletics, and sprinklings of other high or low points he had encountered during his journey. I did the same. It was as if time had not passed. Thirty

The Beginning

years of separate lives didn't faze what was a comfortable, easy conversation. I hadn't laughed that hard in a long time.

When Gene dropped me off at the hotel, I sensed that it wouldn't be the last I would see of him during that visit, and it wasn't. The next night he invited me to attend a high school basketball game he was broadcasting and a homemade meal of spaghetti and meatballs. We had a blast. I was instantly impressed with the ease he had doing his craft. His broadcasting was artistic, his voice lively when needed, while smooth at the same time.

As I headed back to North Carolina the next day, we vowed to keep in touch.

I'd like to say that it was a fairy tale ending, but it wasn't. It was bumpy at first, as we both learned to have a long-distance relationship, knowing that once I sold my house I would be moving closer. It took four months for the house to sell. During that time, we met halfway once, and he visited for several weeks during the spring and summer. We made it work.

When I finally made the move, Gene was there to help me. I drove my three cats to Connecticut in a cargo van, one of them howling the whole way. We turned around less than twenty-four hours later to make the trip back to North Carolina, then drove back north the next day; he drove my Chevy Impala, while I drove my little Mazda Miata. I had been on the road for the third day in a row, but I was excited to start the next chapter.

We had decided to give cohabitating a try. Gene found a great apartment with a breathtaking view of the sunset. Coordinating my stuff getting to Connecticut and closing his bachelor pad after driving over twenty-one hundred miles in three days left me sore and exhausted. When we finally got into the apartment and got the cats out of the kitty hotel, I felt I was where I needed to be. I was happy.

Chapter Two

The Fall

Gene knew that the reason for my return to the place I grew up in was not because I loved the long, harsh winters, high taxes, and congested highways that Connecticut had to offer. I had come back to help my parents in their golden years. At the time, I wasn't sure what that would look like, but I can say it was easy at first.

From the moment I landed in Connecticut, we made the half-hour drive to Old Lyme to visit my parents. Most of the time it was several games of cards, good food, and wine. We laughed a lot and truly enjoyed each other's company most of the time. My aunt joined us some weeks, which added to the fun.

My parents had become a little like hermits. They only ventured out for doctor's appointments or to do the weekly grocery shopping, so I think they looked forward to our weekly visits. It broke up their otherwise mundane lives. We had developed a routine that worked for all of us, and it was one that we truly enjoyed.

On Mother's Day 2011, I got a frantic call from my father. When he returned from church that morning, he walked in to find my mother collapsed on the floor at the bottom of their stairs. He let me know that he had called 911 and that my mother was being transported to the hospital.

The Fall

When I walked into the emergency room, my mother was lying in bed with a huge bump on her forehead and the beginning of an impressive shiner. The doctors were in the process of taking CT scans and X-rays. When the results came back, my mother had a mild concussion and two broken wrists. This was far from the Mother's Day breakfast I had planned.

Four hours later, we left with both her wrists wrapped and plans to return the next day to put metal plates in each of them to stabilize the breaks. Having two broken wrists left her almost helpless. She was hardly able to push herself up and needed help just going to the bathroom.

I took a few days off work to help do what I could. My father would go out to shop while I stayed with Mom, just to give him a break. My mother was never an easy patient, so Dad welcomed my visits. Most days it was like a baton toss as I entered the house and my father left.

It was at this time that I learned that my mother had no tolerance for pain. To manage the pain, the doctors put my mother on oxycodone. I suspected she was taking more than the recommended dose, which was validated when the pharmacy said she couldn't refill her prescription for another two weeks. When I confronted her with this, she did what she always did when someone questioned her, she got angry, but since she could no longer fill her prescription, it was a moot point. Instead, she managed the pain with Tylenol. When I look back, I realize that my mother had been addicted to over-the-counter medication most of her life. If she had a stomachache, she took a pill. If her nose was running, she took a pill. If she couldn't sleep, she took a pill. She did that for as long as I can remember.

After she healed from the broken wrists, things were never quite the same. We would go for dinner and she would have to quickly get up from the table to use the bathroom. She was often not feeling well when I called to check in on them, but we continued to visit on a weekly basis and chalked a lot of her ailments up to old age and the fact that they had settled into a very sedentary life.

When she told me about whatever was ailing her on any given week, my response was always the same. "Have you spoken to your doctor about it?" And the answer was always the same. "No."

During the summer of 2015, I noticed some serious changes that concerned me. I couldn't put my finger on it, but I knew something was wrong with my mother. She had no energy and was very disinterested in life. I figured it was depression, and I did what I could to make a difference. It was during one of their visits that she was sitting on the couch and got up to use the bathroom. As she walked the ten steps from the couch to the bathroom, she peed herself. I could see that her pants were wet. Although she hadn't mentioned anything to me, it appeared that this had happened before. She came prepared with a clean change of underpants and jeans.

Chapter Three

Thanksgiving

Fast-forward to Thanksgiving 2015. We planned our usual get-together. My mom and dad would come to our house for an early afternoon meal, and they would bring my Aunt Paula, who always spent the holidays with us. Gene would do most of the cooking, although when we first got together he let me help much more. I think the kitchen became what he could control after he retired. He had been a boss for so many years that he was struggling with not having anyone to boss around—and Lord knows he wasn't going to boss me around!

My parents arrived by early afternoon, and my mother looked a little wiped out. When I asked her, she said she wasn't feeling that great; the day before had been rough. This didn't alarm me too much, as my mother had become a bit of a hypochondriac in recent years. It became normal when I called and asked how she was to get the response of "I've been better." Of course, each time I asked her what was going on, she would fluff it off as a migraine, a stomachache, or a bad night's sleep. Again, nothing that would alarm me; she'd suffered with these my whole life.

When Gene and I got together, we melded traditions, things we loved about the holidays, and we started some of our own traditions. We started the tradition of making homemade pasta for an appetizer. It was always a hit, and this year was no different.

What *was* different was that two minutes into the first course, my mother started gagging and excused herself from the table. The bathroom was right off the dining room, so I could hear her retching from where I sat. I looked at my father as if to say "WTF," but before I could ask what was going on, she returned to the table.

"Are you okay?" I asked. I could tell she was somewhat embarrassed by what had just happened.

She shrugged her shoulders and said, "I guess so."

I asked her if she had been sick. She said no, that she had been feeling fine, but when she ate, she felt like the food wouldn't go down. I was alarmed.

"Did you call the doctor?" I asked, frustrated.

I knew before I even asked the question what the answer was going to be. Even though my parents were always at the doctor for some test or another, they rarely discussed their overall health.

The rest of the meal went much like the beginning. My mother got up from the table two more times to throw up whatever she tried to eat. Everyone at the table was uncomfortable, and I don't think any of us enjoyed the meal.

After dinner, my mother laid down on the couch, as she often did when she visited, and took a nap. My father was still in the dining room, so I took the opportunity to question him about what was going on.

"I don't know. This just started happening the other day," he said.

"Dad, it isn't normal. She needs to call the doctor," I said, knowing he would have no influence on her making that call.

My mother rarely listened to my father when it came to any kind of advice. In fact, she got downright angry with him if he even hinted at what he thought she should do about anything. So, after sixty years of marriage, he had learned to keep his mouth shut and go with the flow. It just made life easier for him.

Thanksgiving

After my mother woke from her nap, I tried to talk to her. "Listen, Mom. I'm not sure what's going on, but I really think you should call the doctor."

"Nah," she said, "I really don't want to deal with it until after the holidays are over. I'll call and make an appointment after New Year's Day."

And so it was. I called every couple of days to check in, and she always told me it was getting better and I didn't need to worry—but I still did. My parents had formed a habit of telling me what I wanted to hear, unless of course I showed up and asked why one of them was limping or had a bandage on some part of their body. It was probably because when they told me the truth, I usually got mad at the stupid decision they had made that got them hurt.

Like the time my father decided it was a good idea to climb an extension ladder that should have been thrown away years ago to clean the gutters. Because they led such a sedentary lives, both had lost their sense of balance and dexterity. The thought of my father on a two-story ladder cleaning the gutters gave me fifteen new gray hairs and made my blood pressure rise twenty points. My reaction was not without warrant, though, because my father fell from that ladder and landed on the hood of his car, which left a huge dent in it that remains there to this day.

From Thanksgiving until Christmas, my mother kept the truth from me well. It is always a busy time of year, so I couldn't visit as often as normal. So, when I saw the shape my mother was in when she walked in Christmas morning, I gasped. She had visibly lost weight, her skin was very pale, and she had bags under her eyes.

The day was a rerun of Thanksgiving. We ate, she vomited, and then slept. Before they left, I made her promise to call her doctor on January 2. Although annoyed at my insistence, she conceded and promised me she would.

I don't recall now how early it was when I called on January 2, but I know it was early. I could hear the annoyance in my mother's tone as I reminded her to call the doctor as soon as the office opened. She called me later that day to tell me she had an appointment on February 10. I lost it.

"February tenth! Did you tell them that you've been throwing up since before Thanksgiving? That's ridiculous! They can't get you in any sooner?" I was infuriated.

Chapter Four

The Medical System

It's no surprise to anyone who knows me how I feel about our country's medical system. Modern medicine, while it has its place and saved my father and my son's life years ago, has become a system of pill pushers and symptom chasers.

In 2003, I was turned on to a chiropractor after my ex-husband hurt his back. He told me that the chiropractor he was seeing for his back strain was a whole-body doctor, a holistic physician. I was intrigued. My oldest son and I had been struggling for years with asthma. It came on suddenly, with no prior history. My doctor then told me that it was because there were so many trees and flowers in North Carolina that brought it on. I swallowed that explanation hook, line, and sinker. She proceeded to conjure up a cocktail of medicines to help with the symptoms, most of them with harsh side effects.

I had to admit that the thought of being able to control my asthma in a more holistic way was quite a relief. When I started seeing the chiropractor, he explained that everything within our bodies is controlled by our central nervous system, that the nerves up and down our spines are receptors that communicate with our body and brains to keep us healthy. When those nerves are pinched, the signal gets interrupted, much like a tear in an electrical cord. The current doesn't flow properly.

He then asked me if I had ever injured my back or gotten whiplash from an accident. At first nothing came to mind, but then I remembered getting into a fender bender when I was pregnant with my oldest son. At the time I did what most people do when they get whiplash—I took what I could to ease the headache, got some X-rays, and fought through it. I then also remembered a four-wheeler accident I had two years earlier when I was riding in the woods.

He shook his head and explained that my spine was probably out of alignment, and once we corrected that my asthma was likely to disappear. I must admit I was skeptical, but I was willing to give it a try. I visited his office once a week for three months, but I started feeling better after the second week. I consulted with him about getting off the medicine I was on, and he said there was no harm in just stopping whenever I wanted.

I was like a cigarette smoker finally making the decision to quit. I went home and threw all the medicine in the trash, and then I made an appointment for my son. After all, if it worked for me, why wouldn't it work for him?

I won't go into great details about how holistic medicine is far better than modern medicine—there are plenty of well-written books on the topic already—but suffice it to say that once I took the dive, there was no turning back. I even worked through a badly injured bulging disc without having to undergo surgery. It took longer, four months to be exact, and a commitment to healing myself through daily (sometimes three times a day) visits to the chiropractor and a massage therapist, but it worked—and it cost a hell of a lot less than surgery would have!

To this day, I see a chiropractor once a month, and I finally convinced Gene to go too. He had an Achilles tendon problem that he was convinced would require surgery, but after four or five visits, it was getting better. Although he hasn't completely drunk the holistic medicine Kool-Aid, he has seen improvements in his own health.

You can only imagine my passion around the fact that, for years, my parent's doctor had been spoon feeding them prescription after prescription for whatever malady they had. My mother had been on two anti-depressants for years, without one hour of therapy. My research on one of the meds clearly showed that it was to be used in conjunction with psychotherapy *and* should only be used for the short term.

At one time, I counted eighteen different medications that my father was taking. He had type-two diabetes, stemming from a poor diet of processed foods, so he took a pill for that. There were high blood pressure pills, blood thinners, a pill for this, a pill for that, and he too was on the same "short-term" anti-depressant that my mother was on, which he started to take after his parents died. I guessed that his doctor didn't think it was normal for him to be sad after losing both of his parents, so he gave him a pill.

My parents and I bickered for years over their health care. They never questioned why their doctor was putting them on a new medication and continued to take whatever the doctor doled out, unless there was a side effect that didn't sit well. Then they would simply try another med until they got it right.

When my mother told me that she had to wait a month to see her doctor, after telling him that she had been vomiting for three months, I was downright pissed off. After her visit a month later, my blood was boiling. When she called after her visit with the doctor, she told me he wasn't sure what was going on. He explained that she would have to go for some tests, and he gave her yet another prescription. To add fuel to the fire, she told me that the doctor said she wouldn't be able to get the test she needed until March, another month away.

I hung up the phone feeling scared and helpless. How could someone take my mother's condition without a sense of urgency? Why wouldn't her doctor push to rush the tests, knowing she was not able to keep food down? What was the next month going to be like for my mother?

I got in the habit of calling every couple of days to see how she was doing. She was tired all the time, sleeping more hours than not, depressed, and not dealing with her new life well at all. Of course, who could blame her? We still made it down to their house once a week to visit and check in on them, but since eating a meal together was out of the question, our visits were shorter.

In March, my mother finally had the test that her doctor had arranged, an endoscopy. For those unfamiliar with this procedure, it is where they put a camera down the patient's throat and look around to see what they can see. My father had several after the removal of his tumor, which left scar tissue in his throat. The scar tissue would constrict over time, causing food to become lodged in his throat. The doctor would go in periodically and stretch the scar tissue, making it easier for him to swallow. My mother was all too familiar with the process, and a bit anxious.

When she called me later that day, her voice was horse and she sounded exhausted. "They think I have achalasia," she told me.

"What the hell is achalasia?" I asked.

I wasn't surprised when my mother told me that she hadn't asked any questions, didn't know what the prognosis meant, or what the treatment was going to be. What she did tell me was that she had a follow-up visit with her primary doctor on April 18, yet another month away. Keep in mind that we are now five months into my mother not eating properly. At this point, my parents were so used to her vomiting when she ate that she literally ate everything with her head hanging over a trash can. She was losing weight quickly.

Achalasia is a disorder where the muscles in the esophagus do not work correctly. They become constricted and will not push food from the throat into the stomach. My research gleaned that it sometimes happened in people with a history of stomach problems (which my mother had her entire life, with ulcers, etc.) and in older people; she was seventy-nine years old. It all made sense.

While there was no known cure, there were certainly things that could be done, from diet modification, to surgery to remove the damaged muscle, to Botox, which was in its experimental stages as a treatment for it. While I was still definitely concerned, I was hopeful that something could be done to improve my mother's quality of life and make it something she could live with. We had options.

The only thing that stood in the way of deciding which option would work best from my mother was one test. It was a motility test, where my mother would swallow dye while they shoved a camera down her throat to confirm that the muscle was or wasn't working properly. The difference between this test and the previous one was that my mother would have to be awake. She firmly refused. The thought of someone shoving a camera down her throat while she was awake scared the crap out of her, and she was having none of it.

On my next day off after her test, I stopped by for a visit. Their car wasn't in the driveway, but the front door was unlocked. When I walked in, the house was dark and quiet. My mother was sleeping on the pull-out couch in the living room. I nudged her gently so I wouldn't startle her.

***

Let me back up for a minute. What I forgot to tell you is that amongst all this craziness with my mom, I asked Gene if he wanted to get married. We had been engaged for five years, together for seven. I vowed when I got divorced that I would never remarry. I believed that marriage gave couples a reason to misbehave. And Gene knew, even though I had agreed to make the commitment to be his fiancée, it was likely that we would never get married.

Imagine his surprise when I randomly called him early in the morning while I was stuck in traffic on I-95. At the time I was working for a company that made me commute from Middletown, Connecticut, to Darien. On the best day possible, the commute one way was an hour and ten minutes. On most days it exceeded two hours. I had a lot of time to think.

For some reason, that morning it came to me: if I was willing to commit my life to being with this man—and I had—why was I being so stubborn about getting married? After all, I was punishing him for something that happened with a man I never should have married in the first place, so I called him and said we should set a date.

"Have you hit your head? Are you okay?" he said after I asked.

"No, no, I'm fine," I replied.

Once he got over the initial shock, we started planning. We threw several dates around, and finally decided that October 7, 2016 would be our day. It would give us plenty of time to plan, get all the kids on board, and my mother was sure to be better by then.

***

When I saw my mother, she was weak, pale, and looked extremely tired. She got up off the couch where she had been napping and made her way to the bathroom. I sat in the dining room, at the same table where I ate at as a child, and I waited for her. When she came out, she joined me at the table and tried to make light of the situation.

"So, what's new?" she asked.

I looked at her and wanted to cry, but she raised me to be strong in the most extreme circumstances, so I didn't. But what I said next, I said through a choked-up voice.

"Look, Mom, I'm really concerned," I said, trying to keep my composure. "You're losing weight and not eating the right things. We need to put our heads together and make a list of what you can eat—meaning, what will go down—and what foods you need to stay away from. I'm getting married in October, and I really need you to be there."

"I'm not going anywhere," she said emphatically. I wasn't so convinced she was right.

We sat at that table I had sat at a million times before and came up with a list of foods that could get past whatever was going on in her throat and get to her stomach to provide the nutrients her body was so desperately lacking. The list mostly consisted of soft foods—scrambled eggs, ice cream, pudding, toast with no crust, etc. You get the picture.

When my father returned from shopping, I handed him the list and told him to only allow her to eat the foods on that list, that he was to feed her as often as she would allow, and that she could have anything on the list, but nothing else.

I'll tell you that my instructions for my father were very easy in theory, but as you'll recall, neither of my parents were very cooperative when it came to following any direction I gave them.

When I left my parent's house that day, I felt slightly less helpless, but still incredibly concerned that my mother was losing weight and that she still had several weeks before she could see her doctor.

About five minutes into the thirty-minute drive home, I decided to call my mother's doctor. I thought that he needed to know that she was minimizing her current condition, and he needed to know the truth. So, I placed a call to his office and asked to speak to him. I was told he was with patients and was not available. I then proceeded to tell the woman who answered the phone what my concerns were regarding my mother's condition.

"She's weak, tired, and not able to take in food. I am very concerned that I am literally watching my mother die," I explained. She said she would convey the message to the doctor and ask him to call.

You might be thinking that my mother's doctor had no obligation to talk to me about her health. But in 2004, both of my parents added me to their records as the only other person their doctor could talk to about their medical conditions. I thought that would at least spark him to return my phone call, but I was wrong. What it did do is cause him to call my mother and ask her why I was meddling in her medical affairs. He proceeded to tell her to call me to let me know that they had a plan and, without coming right out and saying it, to butt out. I was livid.

After that, I attempted to reach out to her doctor. I called his office again and asked his nurse if he had an email address. Earlier that morning, I had composed an email mapping out my concerns about my mother's health and asking for a partnership with him. I was told he didn't have an email address.

"You mean to tell me he does not have an email address where patients can contact him with questions or concerns? This is 2015! Everyone has an email address," I explained. But my plea fell on deaf ears, and I once again asked him to call me. He never did.

The Medical System

I arranged to take April 18 off from work. I was bound and determined to be an advocate for my mother, who by this time had dropped from 163 pounds to 139. Late on April 17, I received a voicemail from the doctor's nurse inviting me to come to my mother's appointment the next day.

By this time, my mother had lost some control over her bladder. She said she had a couple of accidents but wasn't really concerned. When I asked if she had spoken to her doctor about it, I again knew the answer before I even asked the question. She hadn't mentioned it. The ironic thing is that she didn't seem to even care if she wet herself at home or in public. So, I purchased some panty shields for her. At least if she was wearing one, she wouldn't wet herself in public.

The morning of April 18 was a beautiful spring day in New England. Her appointment was at 11 a.m., so I drove to her house to pick her up. By this time, she had no interest in driving. In fact, she hadn't been out of the house in weeks.

When we got to the doctor's office, I helped her in. She was very unsteady on her feet and needed my arm to keep her upright. Once inside, I led her to the nearest chair and checked in with the nurse. We waited a few minutes and then were called back to the exam room.

While we waited for the doctor to come in, I looked around the room. There were pictures on the wall of some boys in baseball uniforms and formal portraits of a young boy and a girl. They looked like the all-too-familiar school portraits my sons had taken many years ago. There were also framed certificates confirming his status on several medical boards and his diploma from a prestigious medical school.

Maybe I've got this guy wrong, I thought to myself. After all, he was a father, graduated from a good medical school, and appeared to be a pillar in the medical community, but my impression was that he cared very little about my mother's health and that he was arrogant. After all, there were now two instances where he didn't return my calls.

When he entered the room, he introduced himself and shook my hand. He then turned his attention to my mother and asked her how she was feeling.

"I've been better," she said.

That was my mother's pat answer whenever she wasn't feeling better. It didn't surprise me that she answered that way. Then we began to get into the meat of the problem. The doctor explained that the preliminary results of the tests determined that my mother may have achalasia, and to determine the correct course of treatment, she would have to undergo a motility test.

After the doctor finished talking to my mother, I chimed in. "Doctor, my mother is petrified of going through this test. She has flatly refused to allow someone to shove a camera down her throat while she is awake. So, I have a proposal."

I went on. "Is there any way we can admit her to the hospital, have her go through the test under anesthesia, and then if she needs surgery to remove part of her esophagus, she will already be there. Look, it's the only way she'll have this test. And if you're saying she must have it to seal the diagnosis, then we will need to be creative in the way that it's done. We need to have her best interest at heart."

I was encouraged when he agreed to my suggestion. "Let me see what I can do to arrange this, and I will be in touch."

We left there hopeful that something positive was going to happen so that my mother could start eating again and regain her strength. The good news was that people didn't die from this disorder, especially if they modified their diet to soft foods.

***

The Medical System

I have always been a glass-half-full person. When I was growing up, my mother often accused me of looking at life through rose-colored glasses. It was the way I was born, and I am still that way today. I have a way of finding the best in the worst situations. That may be one of the reasons I stayed in a terrible marriage for twenty years. I also learned that we have little control over external sources. We can only control ourselves and how we react to life's bumps and bruises.

When I stood back and looked at my mother's situation, I instantly became anxious. To add fuel to the fire, the motility test that her doctor insisted she have could only be scheduled in July, yet another three months away.

What I did next would have made my Sicilian grandmother proud. I went home and cooked. Since we would have to wait for the test, I needed to get some nutrients in my mother's body. She was becoming a mere shell of herself when this nightmare started.

I started with her favorite soup. It was a Tucson soup loaded with potatoes, Italian sausage, kale, and bacon—tons of flavor, calories, and nutrients. After the soup was done cooking, I took a hand-held mixer and pureed it slightly. I was determined to get as much food into my mom as possible. I made several other dishes I thought she might like, pureed each one, and put them into single-serving containers. This would make my father's life slightly easier, by only having to heat up what she wanted at each meal.

On my way to their house, I stopped at the store and picked up several types of pudding, some Jell-O, ice cream, and some watermelon pops. I grabbed anything that was soft that I thought she might be interested in.

When I arrived at their house with loads of food, I put everything away and sat down at the table with my parents. I also created a spreadsheet so my mother could track what she was eating, and so she would know what was available.

My instructions for my father were simple. "She needs to eat as many times a day as she wants. She needs to eat whatever she wants, whenever she wants," I explained. I had also purchased a couple of different protein drinks that were packed with calories and nutrients. "Make sure she drinks this at least three times a day. It doesn't have to be a big glass, but it will give her the protein she needs to get stronger."

When all was said and done, I felt like it would make a difference. I then proceeded to tidy up the house. My mother couldn't do much to keep things up. In fact, she wasn't doing much at all. Of course, she was weak from malnutrition. Try as he may, my father was no housekeeper. I made a point of stopping by once a week to check in, take my father to the grocery store, tidy up, drop off food, etc.

Of course, I didn't do it alone. Gene was an integral part of the routine. When I wasn't able, he stopped by to check on my parents and bring my father to the store. He always made sure they were set up for the next couple of days and then moved on.

We started attending church during this time. In April, Gene's godson received his holy communion, and we attended the mass at Bishop Seabury Anglican Church. I was so taken with the pastor's sermon that I suggested that we go back. Neither Gene nor I had attended church on a regular basis for years, but there was something about this church that brought me the comfort and strength I so desperately needed.

For the next month, we created a weekly ritual of attending church and stopping at my parents' house on the way home. We would take care of whatever needs they had and then head home. My mother certainly wasn't getting any better. She was getting very discouraged as she waited for the July date to roll around.

The Medical System

After my initial visit to my mother's doctor, I called the office numerous times to discuss my mother's condition. There were a bunch of scheduling hiccups, miscommunication between her primary doctor and various specialists. Appointments were messed up, accidentally cancelled, and communication was a debacle of confusion.

I'll admit there were times throughout the process when I was not nice. I was working sixty hours a week, so I had little time, and less patience, for a medical system that seemed to be so inefficient. After all, these were trained, well-educated, highly paid professionals. I didn't think it was a lot to ask that they be able to accommodate my mother's needs to have this final test under anesthesia—but I was wrong.

The request threw a monkey wrench into the cogs in the medical wheel, and I began to see how rigid the system was. However, I continued to persevere, keeping in mind that this was a world my parents had lived in for years and were comfortable with. After all, it wasn't about me; it was about my mom.

Gene and I stopped by my parents' house in late June after church. I put on a brave face after walking in and seeing my mother's condition. Over the previous week she had become paler and weaker. I watched her come out of the bathroom having to use the walls to steady herself. She stopped in the kitchen to blow her nose, and her pants fell to the ground. She giggled when it happened and reached down to pick them up. Because my mother always wore baggy clothes, I hadn't been able to see how much weight she'd lost. Although I was aware, I didn't really know how much until I saw her standing in the kitchen with her pants around her ankles.

I'll admit I cried for about ten minutes as Gene and I drove home that day. "She's withering away," I said through my tears. "I can't just sit around and watch her die." I felt helpless.

Gene and I talked about the situation for several hours when we got home. I decided that I had to get my mother some much-needed medical attention. On Monday morning, I got up early, placed a call to my mother's doctor, and asked that the doctor return my call.

The nurse from the doctor's office was a very nice woman, but she was ill equipped to deal with my intervention regarding my mother's current condition. I had spoken to her numerous times over the previous months, when appointments were messed up, when I requested that the doctor call me, or even to let her know that my mother's condition was deteriorating. She always had a nervous tone in her voice when we spoke. I'm not sure if it was because I was forceful and matter-of-fact with her, or if that was just her normal state. Quite frankly, I didn't care.

On Tuesday morning, I called the doctor's office again, told the nurse that my mother's condition had worsened, and that I was taking her to the hospital. I then told her that the doctor could be involved or not involved; it didn't matter to me. I was going to pick my mother up at her home and bring her to an emergency room. Within ten minutes of that call, I received a return call that instructed me to take her to a hospital in Hartford that he was affiliated with.

When I brought her into the emergency room, I was, for the first time in months, taken seriously. I told the admitting person that I was concerned that my mother was dehydrated, malnourished, and needed immediate medical assistance. It didn't take a group of specialists to recognize that I was on point with my amateur diagnosis, so they admitted my mother and started pumping her with fluids.

When I tell you that within hours of her getting just a saline solution her color got better, I am not embellishing things. She also started to perk up as she responded to the fluids. They also began to run tests. One of the preliminary tests showed that her potassium levels were very low, primarily because she had not been able to keep food down and her body chemistry was all out of whack.

For those who don't know it, intravenous potassium is very painful, and they were continually pumping that into my mother along with saline. Once they got her somewhat stabilized, I began to ask questions. Since she was already in the hospital, was there a chance they could do the ever-important motility test and whatever procedure was needed to correct the effects of achalasia. In other words, let's get the test done and get whatever it was fixed.

When I brought my mother into the emergency room, there were lots of questions about who I was, and I was told what my legal rights were. Since my mother was present, she gave the hospital staff permission to talk to me, but decisions on medical treatment had to come from my mother. In her weakened state, she was confused at first as to what was happening, so it was imperative that someone be able to make decisions on her behalf. This is when I was introduced to the concept of being my mother's power of attorney. We contacted our attorney.

In a lengthy phone conversation, our attorney explained about the different POAs and suggested that my parents make me their POA for all decisions, medical and financial. He made a trip from his office to visit my parents at the hospital to explain everything, draw up the paperwork and have them sign. This piece of paper would allow me to ask questions, which the doctors were forced to answer. It would become extremely important in the months to come.

My mother was in the hospital for three weeks. During that time there were various tests done, but not the motility test she so desperately needed. They did another endoscopy, an MRI, and a CT scan. I went to the hospital every day to speak with the doctors and determine the next course of action. Each day I was faced with the same answer. They weren't sure what was going on or how to treat it.

It was at this point that the doctors started murmuring about cancer. They were running tests because they firmly believed that what they originally diagnosed as a constriction of the esophagus was cancer. Once that happened, we were scheduled with an oncologist and a radiologist.

I took my mother to both appointments, where we set up a schedule for her to begin treatment. At this point, she was 129 pounds and weak but still able to handle the treatment. So, she opted to undergo chemo and radiation. We went to meet with the radiologist and oncologist. Both specialists were patient and caring, but that didn't ease the fears that my mother and I had.

When we met with the radiologist, they laid out a schedule of treatment that would start in two days. We had scheduled appointments at 10 a.m. each morning for the next six weeks. This would allow me to bring my mother for her treatments each day and be to work by one o'clock. I had arranged everything with my boss, who was very supportive.

"There are bigger things in life. We have to take care of family," he told me when I explained everything to him.

The day before my mother was to have her first treatment, I got a call from the radiologist. "We have met as a collective group and are not completely convinced that your mother has cancer," he explained. "So, we'd like to step back a bit and make sure we're doing what's best for her."

After I hung up the phone with the radiologist, I called my mother and told her the good news. "You don't have cancer," I told her with relief in my voice. "They still aren't sure what's going on, but they have ruled out cancer."

The Medical System

Even with the good news, my mother was still not able to eat. I spoke with another specialist about the options. This was the first time anyone had spoken of a stent. The doctor explained that there was a possibility that they could place a stent in my mother's esophagus that would stretch the constriction and allow food to pass through. He explained that there were some restrictions with the procedure.

First, my mother would have to continue a soft diet. She would no longer be able to eat meat, unless it was ground or pureed. This wasn't a concern, as she was already on a soft diet. He also stated that she could never lie flat on her back again. Because the stint would no longer allow her esophagus to close completely, she could regurgitate her food and choke to death. He suggested we buy a bed wedge.

I'm not sure how you feel about online shopping, but it was our saving grace. Amazon allowed us to buy what we needed, often when we were still in the doctor's office. From bed wedges to bedding to protein drinks, we could have whatever we needed delivered in two days or less.

The procedure to insert the stent would be outpatient surgery. My father, Gene, and I went to the hospital with my mother, but I had to leave early to go to work. Gene called me after the procedure was over and let me know that she came through the surgery fine. His plan was to bring them back to their home in Old Lyme, but I suggested they spend the night at our house, just in case. They agreed.

After they settled in for the evening, Gene called me and updated me on the evening's events. "They both ate dinner. Your mom kept everything down. She seemed all right and went to bed fairly early."

I breathed a sigh of relief. Perhaps we were seeing the beginning of something positive.

The next morning. I rose early, but my parents were already up. My mother was resting on the couch. "How are you feeling?" I asked.

"I've been better," she replied.

"Did you sleep okay?" I asked.

"I did."

I got myself a cup of coffee and offered one to my parents. My mother declined, which was very unusual for her. She loved her coffee. About five minutes into my coffee, my mother got off the couch, staggered her way to the kitchen, and threw up in the sink.

From where I was sitting, I could see that she was vomiting mucus and blood. I was quite alarmed. No one told us that this was normal, so it scared me. We were given a folder filled with paperwork when my mother was discharged the previous day. Amongst the papers was the "just in case" paperwork. There were clear instructions on what to do if we saw blood or if she was vomiting. Both said to call the office immediately.

It was a Saturday morning, so when I called the office, I got the answering service. The nurse explained that she would have the doctor call me within the next fifteen minutes. Fast-forward an hour, and the doctor still had not called. My mother had thrown up four more times. I took matters into my own hands and decided that my mother needed to go back to the hospital. We all climbed in the car, my mother and I in the back seat. She was holding a bag, just in case she needed to throw up.

When we arrived at the emergency room, they took her right away. Turns out that if you say that someone is vomiting blood after a procedure a day earlier, you get noticed. After examining my mother and speaking with the specialist who had inserted the stent, my mother's reaction was not normal, so they decided to admit her for observation. That was mid-July.

The Medical System

Over the next several weeks, the doctors and nurses tried to devise a plan to get my mother on a diet that she could tolerate without vomiting. It didn't appear that the stent was giving her much relief, so they drilled her diet down to liquids, which she seemed to be able to tolerate. They were pumping her full of saline because she was once again dehydrated. They were also giving her potassium through an IV. Turns out that low potassium levels are something that doctors see in third-world countries where people are starving. This news validated my fears; my mother was slowly starving to death.

During her time in the hospital, they did a battery of tests. First, they wanted to verify that the stent had not moved, which would have caused a blockage in her throat. Then they wanted to see if food was flowing from her esophagus to her stomach, which it was. They also ruled out cancer once more, because there were no visible tumors. Even with all these tests, they were still not able to determine why she was unable to eat.

I'll admit that all along the journey, cancer was always in the back of my mind. My mother had struggled with stomach issues her whole life. That and a poor diet pointed directly to cancer. Each time the doctors ruled it out, I was relieved. After all, if it wasn't cancer, it was probably something she could learn to live with.

By this time, she was down to 119 pounds, a mere shell of the person she had been when this nightmare began. Each day that went by without any clear plan of action made me more and more anxious and far less patient.

Now I was having daily conversations with doctors and nurses about what they planned to do to help my mom—most of which were unproductive and frustrating. The doctors needed to consult with each other, the nurses were at the mercy of the doctors, etc., etc.

I learned the hard way that the medical system is filled with roadblocks and speed bumps that make it hard to navigate. The system was ill-equipped to deal with anything other than a textbook diagnosis—and it was not prepared for me to be an advocate for my mother.

If you recall, I mentioned that both my parents had white coat syndrome. They were so convinced that doctors knew everything that was best for them, I had to often remind them that doctors were not gods.

"We've got to figure out a way to get some nutrients into her body," I implored during one hallway conversation with the doctor who was on the floor that day. "I can't continue to watch her wither away."

The saline solution they were dripping into her body through an IV was hydrating her body, which was helping, but it did not provide the calories or nutrients needed for her survival.

Even after the stent was placed in her throat, my mother continued to regurgitate every time she attempted eating. The doctors said that her stomach was spasming because it was not used to taking in food. We tried numerous combinations of foods, and her diet was narrowed down to pudding, Jell-O, rice pudding, and coffee.

The doctors and I started to discuss alternatives. One option was a to insert a feeding tube either in her throat or directly into her stomach. It didn't have to be a permanent solution, but if she opted to go with the tube into her stomach, it would bypass the problem area, her throat. Insertion of the tube would mean her undergoing anesthesia. They would make a small incision in her abdomen and insert the tube. It made perfect sense. Now I just had to convince my mother that it was the right option for her.

The Medical System

It wasn't hard to make her realize it was the only viable option. I told her that it was temporary, and once she gained some weight and got stronger, they would remove it.

Although she was still able to get out of bed with assistance, there was no way my father would be able to care for her at their home in Old Lyme. She needed physical therapy to make her stronger and calories to help her gain back the weight she had lost. Once they inserted the tube, the doctors started talking about releasing her from the hospital. The next step for her was to go into a rehab center where they could monitor her progress, give her physical therapy, and feed her whatever she would eat.

My mother was transported by ambulance to a rehab center down the street from where I lived in Middletown. It was far more convenient than driving to the hospital, but my mother was not happy at all. She was tired of being in the hospital and downright tired of being sick. It was at this point that she became nonverbal. At first, I was convinced she wasn't speaking for fear she would curse someone out. As I think about it now, that's where it began. But as time went on, I just don't think she wanted to talk to anyone.

When the doctor inserted the stent into my mother's throat, he took multiple biopsies of her throat and stomach. By this time, they had completely ruled out cancer, so I didn't understand why they felt compelled to dig further. One specialist I spoke with had reviewed all her records and told me that even though cancer didn't show up on any of the previous biopsies, he had never seen a case like my mother's, where the patient was losing weight so drastically but didn't have a cancer diagnosis.

He also explained that there were two types of stomach cancer. One where there are visible tumors that are easily detected, and the other where the walls of the stomach thicken as the cancer progresses. It was the second type that he was exploring through the biopsies—and he was right.

A week into my mother's stay at the rehab center, I got a call from the specialist while I was at work. "Your mother has gastric cancer," he said. "We'll need to get her to the oncologist as quickly as possible to see what the options are. I'll have their office call you in the next day or so to schedule an appointment."

I hung up the phone and took a deep breath. The last several months had been such a rollercoaster ride. She had achalasia; she didn't have it. She had cancer; she didn't have cancer. The stent was going to work; now it wasn't going to work. Now I was faced with telling her that she had stomach cancer. My heart was broken.

I knew when I hung up the phone that the prognosis was not good. When she was originally diagnosed, she was thirty pounds heavier and much stronger. My fear was that any type of intervention would make her sick and that the cancer was far too advanced at this point for any treatment to be effective.

I left work early that day to tell my mother about the conversation. When I told her she had stomach cancer, she shrugged her shoulders and threw her hands in the air. She became resigned to her illness. I sat on the bed beside her and vowed I was with her all the way, and that wherever this journey took us, we were going together.

Moments later my phone rang. It was the receptionist from the oncologist's office. She said they had an appointment at 10:30 the next morning and that the doctor wanted to see my mother right away. I told her we would be there and hung up the phone. I walked back into my mom's room and told her about the appointment, trying to be cheerful and positive. She gave me a thumbs-up.

The Medical System

Gene and I talked later that night, and I voiced my concerns about her going through chemo. "There's no way that her body can handle the poison. She'll die from the treatment, not the disease."

He and I were all too familiar with this scenario, as it had happened to his father in 2012 when he underwent chemo and radiation for lung cancer. His body was far too weak to handle the effects of the poison by the time they started treatments. He probably could have lived another year or two before the cancer got him without the treatment, but we'll never know.

The next morning, I got to the rehab center in enough time to help my mother get dressed. She had lost several things while there, including a religious medal she had worn around her neck for years. My grandparents brought it back on one of their many trips to Italy. One day when I came to visit, she motioned to her neck and I saw it was gone. Fortunately, my grandparents brought one back for me at the same time, so the next day I brought her mine and hung it around her neck. She held the medal in her hands and smiled. I was sure it brought her comfort.

She had also lost the set of clothes I brought for her the day after she arrived. Even though she never wore them, they had disappeared. After that, I was careful not to leave anything that she didn't want to part with forever. I brought a set of clothes and helped her get dressed. My father and Gene waited in the hallway. The rehab center let us use a travel wheelchair to transport her from her room to the car. By this time, she could not walk without assistance, and there was no way she could make it to the car.

We got to the oncologist's office thirty minutes early. Gene had even taken the scenic route to get there. The wait in the lobby seemed like an eternity. When her name was finally called, my mother, father, Gene, and I piled into the tiny examining room. While we waited for the doctor to come in, my mother nodded off. Just the short fifteen-minute trip had exhausted her.

There was a soft knock on the door, which opened slowly. The oncologist walked in, greeting us with a warm smile. She was of Indian descent, and I guessed she was in her mid-thirties. I surmised this because she had previously spoken of her two sons, who were nine and ten. My mother and I had seen the same doctor back in June when she was originally diagnosed with cancer. She was a soft-spoken woman who had gentle eyes. From the certificates, newspaper articles, and various forms of prestigious recognition that hung on the walls, I knew that she was tops in her field—not to mention that I liked her presence from the moment she walked in the room.

"Mrs. Lorello, how are you feeling?" she asked, holding my mother's hand in hers.

My mother did what she normally did those days. She shrugged her shoulders and put her hands up in the air in resignation. I could see from the expression on her face that she was alarmed that the woman sitting in the wheelchair was indeed the same woman she had seen only months earlier. She and I had a silent conversation with crinkled foreheads, eyes darting back and forth, a sad smile from me, and some deep breaths.

"Let's look at things," she said, turning back to the computer screen.

She looked over the notes while we all waited for her to speak. When she finally spoke, she spoke to me directly, in a way that she knew I would understand but that neither my father nor mother would comprehend. What she told me was that my mother had stage-four gastric cancer. She also told me that any type of treatment would only prolong her life, that it would not cure the cancer. She also said that the treatments would be very hard on her, given her current condition.

Once she was convinced that Gene and I understood, she turned to my mother. "Mrs. Lorello, you have stomach cancer." She took my mother's hand and looked into her eyes.

My mother rolled her eyes as if to say, "Been there, done that."

Then the doctor went over the options. She was recommending chemo and radiation but was realistic in letting my mother know that the cancer was advanced and that any treatment would only prolong the inevitable. She said that the decision was up to her; she would honor whatever course of action my mother decided. Then she stepped away from my mother's wheelchair.

I was quite choked up at this point but kept it together. After all, my mother had just been given her death sentence. I stepped over to where she was sitting in the wheelchair and knelt in front of her. "What do you think?" I asked.

Once again, she shrugged her shoulders.

"Do you want to know my thoughts?" I asked. She nodded her head yes. "If you go with the chemo, it's likely to make you very sick. It's not going to cure you; it will simply slow the cancer down, but whatever time you have left, you could be very sick, which doesn't make much sense to me, because you're going to die either way.

"Here's what we know, we know that you're going to die, and so are each of us. We also know what you're going to die from; not many of us know that, which probably isn't much of a comfort, but what we don't know is when. It could be tomorrow, it could be a year from now, or five years from now. So, how about we make the most of whatever time you have left and not do it under the influence of drugs and poison?"

Her eyes never left mine during my little speech. I felt we were connected at the soul. I knew she trusted me implicitly, and she agreed that my suggestion was the best course of action. I hugged her tightly and told her I would be with her every step of the way. We were in this together.

I turned to the doctor, who said she would write the prescription for hospice care and get the ball rolling. We wheeled my mother out of the office, my eyes filled with tears, knowing that this was the beginning of the end.

SUBSCRIPTION ORDER

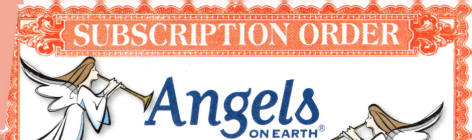

Angels ON EARTH®

Mail this card to start or renew your own subscription ...or give a friend a gift!

Send no money—we'll bill you later!

(Fold and detach at perforation and mail card below.)

☐ **1 YEAR** $18.00* plus $1.95 delivery
$20.95 Canadian/$25.95 Foreign

☐ **2 YEARS** $33.00* plus $2.95 delivery
$37.95 Canadian/$47.95 Foreign

YOUR NAME (Please print)

Address _____ Apt. _____

City _____ State _____ ZIP _____

E-mail _____

PREFERRED SUBSCRIBER

☐ Include my own subscription.

Send a gift and a gift card in my name for: ☐ **1 Year** ☐ **2 Years**

GIFT TO (Please print)

Address _____ Apt. _____

City _____ State _____ ZIP _____

guideposts.org/aoe

*Sales tax added where applicable.

AOEJ2031IDA1

Preferred Subscriber Guarantee

1. We guarantee that you may cancel your subscription(s) at any time upon request and that you will receive a prompt refund on any unserved issues.
2. We guarantee to continue your gift subscription(s) at the then current rate for as long as you wish, without interruption, unless you instruct us to stop.
3. We guarantee if you include your own subscription we will also provide continuous service at the then current rate for as long as you wish.
4. Send no money now. As a Preferred Subscriber, a gift card will automatically be sent in your name every year (on receipt of payment) to the person named on the reverse side.

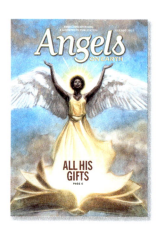

Thank you for your support!

(Fold and detach at perforation and mail card below.)

AOEJ2O3LIDA1

BUSINESS REPLY MAIL
FIRST-CLASS MAIL   PERMIT NO. 329   HARLAN IA

POSTAGE WILL BE PAID BY ADDRESSEE

NO POSTAGE NECESSARY IF MAILED IN THE UNITED STATES

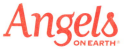

PO BOX 5812
HARLAN IA 51593-3312

Chapter Five

The Hospice Angels

Navigating in a world with words like palliative care, hospice care, and home healthcare was something I had never experienced before, but I learned quickly.

When we brought my mother back to the rehab center that afternoon, I let the nurses know she had cancer and that we would be taking her home under hospice care (not that I really knew what that meant at the time). The main nurse suggested I set up a meeting with the social worker to plan to take my mother home. I set up an appointment for the very next morning.

By this time my mother had all but shut down. She was no longer speaking to anyone, and on the rare chance that she did, she was angry and caustic. I visited her every day in the rehab center, but we rarely spoke. We held hands a lot. She slept, and I watched her. I found comfort in being there to hold her hand and smile at her when she woke up.

Every day I would try to get her to eat something, but she had no appetite and hated the food there. She didn't hate just the food, she hated everything about it. I told her that once everything was arranged that she would be getting out of there to come to my house in Middletown.

It was then she said, "But I want to go home," meaning their house in Old Lyme.

"Mom, there's no way that Dad can take care of you. You should come to my house so that the three of us can care for you." She rolled her eyes in protest, but she knew I was right.

The next few days were a flurry of activity. I met with the social worker at the rehab center the next morning. She had already started the wheels in motion. They received the prescription from the oncologist to place my mother on hospice care. I learned that it was a medical doctor who makes the decision whether someone can go on hospice care or not. Since my mother had the blessing—if that's what you can call it—from her oncologist, the rest was just a bunch of paperwork.

We arranged for a hospital bed to be brought in to replace the queen bed we currently had in our downstairs bedroom. Our home was perfectly laid out for my mother to come live with us. We had one bedroom and a full bathroom on the first floor, and two more bedrooms and a bath on the second floor. We removed the existing queen bed and bought my father a twin bed, which was put in the same downstairs room with my mother. He had been already living with us for the last couple of months so that it was easier on us for him to visit my mother. I felt it was important for him to spend as much time as he could with her, since we didn't know how much time she had left.

The last piece of the puzzle was the feeding tube that was inserted in my mother's stomach. She couldn't take in much orally, but the feeding tube was providing her with much-needed calories and nutrients. What I was about to learn is that a feeding tube is not part of palliative care. Hospice care is primarily pain management and feeding someone artificially was not covered.

"We can't send her home with the feeding tube," the doctor at the rehab center explained. "We'll have to remove the tube before we send her home."

I looked at my mother. "Now it's all up to you. If you don't eat, it's going to go downhill quickly." She shrugged her shoulders. All she wanted was to go home, and I think she would have cut off one of her feet if I told she had to.

Within minutes, they shut off the feeding machine, clamped off the tube, and the doctor said he would remove it in the morning. When I got there the next morning, the feeding tube was still in. When he came in the room, I asked him why it wasn't out. He said he met resistance when he tried to remove it and wanted to consult with one of the doctors at the hospital. He said there was no harm in the tube staying in, but that he did notice that some of her stomach acid was leaking out of the hole and we needed to keep an eye on it. He gave us some ointment and bandages to take home with us.

It was the Tuesday after Labor Day 2016 when we were finally able to bring her home. It was early afternoon, and we got her settled into the hospital bed in the downstairs bedroom. Gene had to go to work that afternoon to broadcast a game, but I was home in case she needed anything.

Soon after he left, she said she needed to use the bathroom. Although the rehab center had deemed her incontinent, they were still getting her up to use the bathroom when she asked, and they encouraged us to do the same. She was in an adult diaper at this point, but when she asked to go to the bathroom, I assisted.

After she was finished, I bent over to wipe her bottom, and something odd happened. She went limp and all her weight was on me, which felt like two tons. I sat her back on the toilet and she was hunched over. I panicked. She was unresponsive and her bowels let loose. I yelled for my father to bring me my cell phone and called 911.

I explained to the 911 operator that my mother had recently been diagnosed with cancer and that something had just happened. The woman asked if she was breathing, which she was, but I told her she was unresponsive. My father was just outside the bathroom looking more scared than I had seen him my whole life. The operator asked me a few more questions, and by this time I could hear the ambulance in the background. As they were pulling up to the house, she was starting to come around.

My house was built in the 1940s and the bathrooms are very small. It was already crowded with just my mother and me in there. Add in a husky EMT, and it was like a sardine can—and from my mother's blow out, it smelled just as bad. The driver helped me clean her up as best we could and transported her to the gurney. They wrapped up and began to take vitals. At this point, she was awake and aware. If fact, I'm sure if she could have, she would have asked what the hell had just happened.

Although she seemed okay, I asked them to transport her to the hospital to be checked out. By this time, Gene was home from work, only to find an ambulance in the front of the house. After they wheeled her out, my father, Gene, and I hopped in the car for the mile drive to the hospital. When we got there, she was already in a room and they were taking her vital signs. When the nurse came in, I introduced myself and explained that I was my mother's POA.

I gave her the abridged version of my mother's recent medical history and a synopsis of what happened in the bathroom. She took my mother's vitals, and at first glance everything looked okay. I also told her that my mother was on hospice care. From my explanation, she guessed that my mother had a seizure. She said they could run a bunch of tests to see what damage was done, if any, but she also explained that further testing was not in keeping with hospice care. Therefore, we got her dressed and took her home.

The next morning, after a restless night's sleep, I got a call from the hospice social worker. She asked if she could stop by the house for a visit. I was already impressed. My mother hadn't been home for twenty-four hours and we were already seeing action. I then got another call from the man who was to be my mother's nurse, saying he would be stopping over later that day to evaluate my mother.

Jan, the social worker, arrived thirty minutes after she called. She pulled up in a little sports car with a rag top. When she came to the door, she held out her hand and introduced herself. She had a warm smile and a gentle way about her. I liked her instantly.

She came in and introduced herself to my father, who was sitting on the couch, to Gene, who was busy in the kitchen, and settled in to chat with me. She opened her laptop and began to ask questions for some type of electronic form she was filling out. At first her questions were of a practical nature. What religion did my mother practice? Did she have a living will? Was she an organ donor? And so on. Then Jan got into questions that were a little more personal—her favorite food, favorite music, and the like. I had to elicit some help from my father for answers to some of her questions. It was then that I realized that I knew my mother better than he did, even though they had been married for over sixty years.

After we answered Jan's questions to the best of our ability, she settled in to teach us how to navigate the hospice system. When I explained what happened the night before that landed my mother in the emergency room, she let us know that going forward that that would change.

"If something like that happens again, don't call 911. Here is the number you'll call in case of an emergency." She handed me a refrigerator magnet that contained the number for the hospice floor. "The nurse will be able to determine how to handle any emergency that comes up."

Jan went on to explain what hospice care was all about. From my limited experience, I knew that hospice got involved when people were terminally ill with no hope of survival. Now, that's not to say that there aren't cases where people survived, but it wasn't the norm. So, some of what she explained I already knew. Things like my mother would have a regular visit from a nurse to check her vitals and assess her condition, but what I didn't know was that she could have regular visits from a spiritual healer, she could get massages, a social worker would be assigned to her, and the list went on.

I was impressed. This part of the medical system seemed so much more about the person than the process. It felt personal, caring, and calm, a far cry from the cold system we had entered in February. These people really seemed to care.

Jan chatted with us for quite some time. She asked my father about their marriage, and to my surprise he was quite candid with her. It was as if he was purging his feelings. "She has not been an easy woman to live with," my father confessed, "but we stuck it out, and here we are today."

Jan listened with great patience.

"If she would only eat some more, she could get better," he said.

Even though my father won his battle with cancer years ago, my mother's cancer was something he didn't understand. For him, an operation and several weeks of chemo and radiation had eradicated his cancer, and it never returned. Therefore, he thought if they operated on my mother that the same would be true for her. We tried to explain that it was a different set of circumstances, but he wasn't buying it. In fact, he thought we should try to contact the same doctor who had operated on him all those years ago. In his small little piece of the world, it made perfect sense.

I poured Jan a cup of coffee. My father excused himself and retreated to the dining room where he had set up shop with his coloring books.

***

When my father retired, he didn't know what to do with himself. He batted around the idea of getting a part-time job pumping gas at the local station. It was walking distance from their house, so it would have been a perfect. He never pursued it, but he did take up the hobby of doing paint-by-number projects. Granted, it's not the most desirable art form, but it kept him busy and he liked it. My mother used to complain that all my father did was paint. He would suck his teeth and roll his eyes.

In the last year, he had given up painting. I think it was because he had painted every kit he found interesting. Our family gave him paintings for every holiday. The finished products were stacking up. Once a year he would donate them to the local church's annual tag sale. I'm not sure if any of them sold, but it made him feel good to donate them. I had my own special collection, most of which were tucked away in my attic. His paintings were too sterile for my liking, but I would never hurt his feelings, so when he gifted one to me, I accepted it as if it were a rare Picasso. In fact, we used to kid him about his painting, and my mother had a pet name for him.

"Hey, Picasso, show Barbara your latest masterpiece," she would say whenever I came to visit.

When he gave up painting, I introduced him to adult coloring books. He seemed to enjoy this new hobby, so we did as we always did, we inundated him with coloring books. He spent hours coloring in those books. I honestly think he was trying to solve the problems of the world.

My father was raised to be a worrier. His mother was a worrier, so she taught him well. He never understood the concept of controlling what you could control and giving the rest up to God. He worried about everything. He worried about my sister and brother. He couldn't understand why they never called. He worried about me, although I tried to not give him a reason to. He worried about my mother, his sister, the cat, his neighbors. You name it, he worried about it. I think painting, and now coloring, allowed him to tune out his worries for a little while.

***

Over coffee, Jan and I began to speak candidly in my father's absence. I told her what had happened over the last several months, how my father was living with us, their history of mental illness, etc.

"Through all this, you seem very centered," she said, somewhat surprised.

"I have my faith," I explained. "I believe in a higher purpose and that God has a plan for all of us. I know that each of us will reach the end of our life here on earth, but that we go to a better place, one where there is no pain or sorrow, only joy and love."

Jan nodded her head in agreement.

"So, my job now is to make whatever time she has left here as good as it can be. I want to care for her, love her, and let her die with dignity when the time comes. It's important that she is as comfortable as she can be."

The Hospice Angels

We chatted for some time as we drank our coffee. I talked about my children; Jan talked about hers. She had recently attended her daughter's wedding. You could tell she was proud of her daughter. It was written all over her face.

As I walked her to the door, we hugged, and I knew that Jan would be a sense of strength for me in the coming months—as would many people.

The next morning, I got a call from Zack, the man who would become my mother's nurse. He said he would be coming by later that morning. When I told my mother that her nurse was a man, she cringed. I had a feeling that the thought of a male nurse was beyond her narrowmindedness. Men were supposed to be doctors, not nurses. But as always, she shrugged her shoulders and threw her hands in the air.

When Zack arrived, he parked his truck on the opposite side of the street from our house. I went to check to make sure my mother was awake. Gene answered the door when he knocked, and I could hear them introducing themselves from the other room. When I came out to the living room, I introduced myself, and he asked if he could sit on the couch.

I found it interesting that when Jan visited the day before, she had placed a sterile pad underneath her before she sat on the couch. Zack did the same. He opened his laptop and pulled up my mother's file. We went over the notes that Jan had taken the day before. Zack added a few notes of his own and asked if he could examine my mother.

My mother was watching TV when we stepped in. Before they started living with us, my oldest son lived with us for a while. He felt that mounting a 46-inch television in the small bedroom was the right thing to do. I thought it was overkill, but it wasn't my money. When he moved out, he decided to leave it—for the small price of $150. Gene loved to watch it while he was walking on the treadmill I had bought him a few years earlier. Now my mother could enjoy watching her favorite shows while she was resting. She loved watching *The Big Bang Theory* and the Game Show Network.

I introduced my mother to Zack. She seemed indifferent. He shook her hand and asked her how she was feeling. She gave him a thumbs-up. Zack asked her if she was in any pain. She pointed at the remainder of the feeding tube that was on the left side of her abdomen.

It had only been a couple of days since the rehab doctor tried to remove it unsuccessfully, but in that time, it had started looking raw and was oozing a yellowish substance. He was very concerned and said that the liquid was stomach acid that was burning and eating away at her flesh. We were cleaning and dressing the wound three times a day, but it was getting worse. I was concerned that it was infected, but it wasn't. Zack still wanted the feeding tube taken out so she would be more comfortable. He said he would put orders in to have it done at the hospital. That was on Thursday.

If you have no experience with the medical system, I can tell you that it is a four-day work week. However, it isn't for the hard-working nurses and aides who make up much of the work force, the people who are really helping patients. That four-day work week pertains to the doctors and surgeons. From my observation, Fridays are reserved for emergencies, those patients who may not make it through the weekend without some type of medical intervention.

My mother was not an emergency; she was just extremely uncomfortable. Her nurse called on Friday to tell me that the tube would not be removed until next week.

By Sunday, the flesh around the tube opening was flaming red and angry looking. Each time we touched it she winced in pain. When the nurse stopped to see her on Monday and saw the condition of the wound, he went into action. While I was at work later that day, he called to tell me that they would admit her to the hospital the next day. I had been under the impression they would remove the tube through an outpatient procedure, but they wanted to remove it surgically. They felt it would be less painful for her.

Zack went on to tell me that they would pick her up by ambulance the next day, do the procedure, and then monitor her overnight. I was concerned about her undergoing anesthesia in her compromised state, but he reassured me that everything would be fine.

That morning before I went to work, I reassured my mother that everything would be okay. It would be a quick trip in and out, and she would be much more comfortable once the tube was removed. Once again, she trusted me. I told her I would stop by to see her after work but that it would be very late.

Throughout the day, Gene kept me updated through text messages. After the ambulance came, he and my father had lunch and then went to visit my mother. She was at Middlesex Hospital on the seventh floor, the hospice floor. By Gene's description, he walked out of the elevator and walked into Shangri-La. He had never seen anything like it before and may never see anything like it again. He said the floor was beautiful. There were serene colors on the wall, beautiful artwork on the walls, soft lighting, and soothing music everywhere. And it smelled like fresh-baked brownies. It was an awakening of the senses.

It looked nothing like any hospital floor he had ever been on. When he found my mother's room, which was near the elevator on the right-hand side, he and my father walked in. He told me that the room was spacious and that everyone was nice. Since I was still working full-time, Gene had the task of bringing my father to visit my mother. They had gone to see her every day during her previous times in the hospital, and twice a day when she was at the rehab center. Now they were seeing her again in a hospital room, but one that was so different that it made Gene feel at ease.

He updated me later in the day to let me know that the surgeon had not been in to see my mother. This was no shock and was par for the course in the medical world. My mother was annoyed, but she was going to be spending the night anyway, so it didn't matter that much.

Later that night I stopped by the hospital on my way home from work. It was after eleven o'clock, so I had to enter through the emergency room. I asked the woman at the desk how to get to the hospice unit.

"Follow the hallway to the elevators on the right. It's on the seventh floor."

I entered the elevator and pushed the button for the seventh floor; it lit up. The elevator started moving and didn't stop until we got to the seventh floor. The hospital was all but deserted at that time, so there wasn't the normal stop and go of the busy hospital elevators. When I stepped out of the elevator, I paused for a moment. Gene was right. This was like no other hospital floor I had ever seen. Now, granted, it was the middle of the night, so there wasn't much movement, but there were no sounds of machines pumping or beeping. There weren't tons of people in the hallway. It was quite peaceful. I recall telling a friend later that if it weren't for the dying piece, I wouldn't mind living on that floor.

I walked down the hall, peeking into each room to see if I could find my mother. After the second room, I began to feel weird, like somehow I was invading people's privacy. I saw a nurse talking to a couple a few doors up and walked over to them. They were finishing their conversation, and I heard the nurse say, "It won't be long now." My heart sank. I didn't know when, but I knew someone would be saying those same words to me soon.

Once the couple walked off, I introduced myself to the nurse and asked where my mother's room was. She pointed to the room just up the hall from where we were standing. She told me to stay as long as I liked. I walked in and stopped to take it all in.

My mother was sleeping. I could hear her quiet snore in the otherwise silent room. She looked peaceful. She was lying on her side, with pillows behind her to keep her there. She had been in bed for so long in the hospital and rehab center that they were concerned about bed sores. She was wearing a pink nightgown, not the normal johnnie that she had worn during her previous hospital visits. On her bed was a beautiful white afghan decorated with crocheted red roses. The lights were dim but not out. I took the chair next to her bed and sat there looking at her. She was the most beautiful I had ever seen her. It brought tears to my eyes.

She was always able to sense when I was in the room, and this time was no different. She stirred and opened her eyes. I wiped my tears away, gave a brave smile, and took her hand. She just smiled.

"How are you doing?" I asked. I got the usual thumbs-up. "Good. They said they're going to take that nasty tube out in the morning, and you'll be home in time for afternoon coffee." She rolled her eyes. She too had become accustomed to the hurry-up-and-wait timing of the medical system.

Her eyes started getting heavy. "Look, I'm going to go home and let you rest. I have to work in the morning, but I'll be home by dinner, and I'll see you then."

I kissed her forehead and told her I loved her. She was asleep again before I was out of the room. As I waited for the elevator,

I took a deep breath. It was more to gain my composure than anything, but when I did I got a whiff of fresh-baked brownies, it made me smile to think that with all the bad stuff happening in the world, all the death and destruction, if we could all just bake some brownies, the world would be a much better place.

The next day I went to work before anyone else was awake. The retailer I work for opens very early, which requires me to rise at 3:15 in the morning at times. Gene sometimes gets up with me, to what purpose I never quite understood, other than the fact that he wanted to get me ready for work. It was something he did in his first marriage that his ex-wife never appreciated, but I certainly did.

This morning he opted to stay in bed, so the house was quiet. I went about my ritual of getting ready and was off to work by four. At this point I was driving my parents' car. They owned a smaller car that was hard for Gene to drive, and since he and my father were driving back and forth to the hospital daily, I wanted them to be comfortable in my bigger car. I must admit I didn't like driving their car at first. It was small, and I felt vulnerable on the busy interstate with all the trucks. I eventually got used to it though.

Later that morning I got a text from Gene. "Call me when you can. Not an emergency." It wasn't the first time I'd received a text message from him like that, nor would it be the last.

I stepped off the floor and dialed his number. By the time I returned his call, it was eleven o'clock in the morning. "The surgeon hasn't even been in to see your mom," he said. "She's getting really agitated and wants to go home."

"Well, tell her she's not going anywhere until they get that thing out of her stomach and to relax," I said. "Tell her I'll be there in a couple of hours." I hung up the phone and asked my boss if I could leave.

"There are bigger things than this company." He always said the same thing every time I needed to come in late or leave early.

On my way home, a forty-minute drive in most cases, Gene called again. I answered the phone. "What's up?"

What he told me next sent chills up my spine and made me a bit nauseous.

"Well, the surgeon was just in to see your mom," he said with a tone in his voice that I knew there was something else coming.

"And?" I asked, knowing I would have to ask to get the rest of the story.

"She yanked the tube out of your mother right in the room," he said, chuckling.

"You're kidding!" I yelled. "WTF."

He went on the explain that a female surgeon stopped in to see my mother, looked at her condition, and determined that she would not be able to undergo any type of sedation. She checked with the surgeon who originally put in the tube to determine what kind it was. When she hung up, she said it would be a simple thing to do. She instructed Gene to hold my mother down, and before anything else was said, she yanked the tube out. Gene said my mother yelled out in pain, but it was over in seconds and the tube was finally gone.

When I got to the hospital thirty minutes later, my father and Gene were still there. My mother was resting comfortably, my father was dozing in the chair, and Gene was playing on his iPad. We both became addicted to a puzzle game during the time my mother became sick. It made it much easier to pass the time while visiting and waiting for doctors.

Gene brought me up to speed on what happened after the surgeon left. Once over the initial shock, my mother instantly felt more comfortable. The surgeon told Gene we would need to continue to clean and dress the wound, but that it should heal over within the next couple of weeks. He then informed me that they would be keeping her overnight for observation. I looked over at mom, and she rolled her eyes, shrugged her shoulders, and threw her hands in the air. We all laughed.

I was off from work the next day, so I was at the hospital early. I left Gene and my father at home having coffee and watching the *Today Show*. It was their morning ritual. They often took advantage of my time off so that I could go visit mom and give them a break.

When I got to the hospital, my mother was sleeping. I spoke to the nurse about when she was coming home. "We'll transport by ambulance around 2:30. The nurse will call you when she leaves the hospital," she said. "Your nurse will be in to check on her tomorrow morning at home, but in the meantime, if you need anything you have our number."

Mom was waking when I returned to her room, so I stayed to visit with her for a while. She was drowsy but comfortable and wanted to go home. I explained how the day was going to work but left the timeframe very vague. I didn't want her to get anxious if things took longer than expected.

I left the hospital around noon to take care of some errands. My time off the past few months had become a balancing act of grocery shopping, laundry, doctor's appointments, paying bills for both me and my parents, and then carving out a little time to spend with Gene. I became very good at the balancing act, but I had very little down time during those months.

I finished shopping and was home in time for my mother to arrive from the hospital. I busied myself with chores that needed to get done around the house. It was close to 2:30, and I still hadn't heard from the hospital. This didn't alarm me at all, so I continued puttering.

When 3:00 rolled around, I started to get nervous. I hadn't heard from anyone, and my mother still had not arrived. I thought

I would give them another thirty minutes or so and then I would call the hospital. At 3:25 my cell phone rang. I didn't recognize the number, but it was the local area code, so I picked up.

"Hello," I said.

"Hello, is this Barbara?" the voice on the other end asked.

"It is," I replied.

"This is Jim from Hunter Ambulance. We've transported your mother, Elizabeth, to Boughton Road in Old Lyme, and no one seems to be at home," he explained.

I laughed out loud. "You weren't supposed to bring her to Old Lyme," I explained. "You were supposed to bring her to my house in Middletown. I live a mile from the hospital." He chuckled nervously.

I gave him my address, and he said they would be there in thirty minutes. I asked if my mother was okay, and he said she was comfortable, which I didn't believe. Riding in an ambulance is far from comfortable.

It was slightly after four o'clock when the ambulance pulled up in front of my house. I opened the front door and waited for them to pull my mother's gurney out of the back.

"Well, hello there," I called from the door as they lowered the legs on the gurney. "How was your ride?"

By this time, I'm sure you can guess what she did. She rolled her eyes, shrugged her shoulders, and threw her hands in the air. The EMT drivers apologized for the confusion and brought my mother to her room. Once they transferred her to the hospital bed and made sure she was comfortable, they left. I got her some water; I could tell she was thirsty. After all, she had been on the road for a few hours by this point.

From there, we settled into a routine. My mother was no longer able to hold her own weight, so any time she wanted to get out of bed, Gene had to help. Watching them work together was like watching two people dance. We would lift her to a sitting position and scoot her to the edge of the bed. Gene would then lean down, and she would wrap her arms around his neck. On the count of three, she would stand, pivot, and back into her wheelchair. He would cover her legs with a blanket and push her wheelchair backwards from the bedroom.

"Weeee!" she would say in a high-pitched voice. It made us laugh every time.

Keep in mind that for the last several months my mother was pretty much nonverbal, and for those who knew my mother, that was a miracle. She had been a very opinionated person who voiced her opinions openly her entire life—even when no one wanted to hear them. The thought of her not talking was so completely foreign to those who knew her that some didn't believe me.

However, there were a few things she said often during that time. For instance, she told me she loved me often. She was grateful and said "thank you" often. That was about it, except for two other times during the day. Each morning when she woke up, and late each afternoon, she would smile real big and say in a high-pitched voice, "Coffee?"

This meant she wanted to get out of bed, be wheeled out to the living room, and join us for morning and afternoon coffee. Gene would make a fresh pot of coffee for her, we'd set up a TV table beside her, change the channel to her favorite show, and plop her in the middle of the living room. She was always welcome to stay as long as she liked.

When we first brought her home, she would sit with Gene and my dad (and me on my day off) for several hours before getting tired. She would often try to eat something too. Gene would go through a restaurant-length menu full of options that she could eat. We decided it didn't matter what she ate, she just needed to eat. After all, with the feeding tube gone, the only nutrients she was getting was what she was eating, which wasn't much. He tried to get her to eat several times a day. Some days he was successful, and some days he wasn't, but whatever she wanted, he would cook, day or night.

It was sometime shortly after she got home from her hospice stay that Gene gave her a nickname. By this time, I had tried several on for size myself. Elizabeth was my favorite. I felt that calling her Elizabeth gave her some dignity. It was more formal, more respectful. But it was the name that Gene came up with that stuck; he called her Toots.

Every time he walked into her room he said, "Good morning, Toots," or "Hello, Toots," or "Are you ready, Toots?" He also called her "Lady," but I liked Toots the best.

As I wrote previously, the hospice part of the medical profession was a breath of fresh air after what we had gone through in the past months. My mother's nurse was great, the social worker was great, and the home health aides were amazing. I'll be honest, though, the home health aides were the part my mother liked the least, but they were the most important to Gene and me.

My mother had become incontinent, and after the episode she had the night she came home from the rehab center, I never tried to take her out of bed alone again. Along with that comes the distinct smell of urine anywhere the person is. Having someone come in three times a week to bathe her was very important to us.

When we originally talked to my mother about coming to live with us, we made it clear that she would have to cooperate. She would need to eat as much as she could and try to be as pleasant as she could under the circumstances, but when it came to someone bathing her, someone she didn't know, she fell short.

At first she cooperated. She didn't like it, but when I told her it helped Gene and me and that she needed to stay clean, she gave in. She was a very private person, and the hospice agency's system did not allow for the same person to come each time. It didn't take long for her to grow tired of strangers washing her body. Sometimes I think she faked sleeping so she didn't have to get a bath.

These women are angels sent directly from God. They took very good care of my mother. They bathed her, washed her hair, put lotion on her, and massaged her feet. It was one less thing we had to do, and it was greatly appreciated.

With incontinence comes the obvious—adult diapers that need to be changed. Gene and I got into a routine with this chore too. Every morning, while the coffee was brewing, we would go in to change my mother. Most mornings she was awake and waiting for us. I would lean over, give her a kiss, and say good morning. I'd ask her if she slept well, to which she usually gave me a thumbs-up. Then I would change her. Gene and I became synchronized at this process. Scissors to cut the sides of her diaper, wipes to clean her up, a trash bag to put everything in, and a clean diaper for her. We all worked together. Mom even did her part, lifting her hips so we could get the new diaper on her. A couple of times she looked me in the eye and asked me if I was tired of doing all this. I told her I would do it for the rest of my life if I could, and I meant it.

My mother had changed from the caustic, callus person she had been most of my life, to a grateful, loving person. I would have done anything to heal the cancer that was eating her body, so that she could stay here on earth. I knew that wasn't likely, but I wanted to make sure she didn't feel guilty. After all, I moved back to Connecticut to help them as they aged. However, I must admit that I never thought I was going to help them die.

Chapter Six

The Wedding

My mother moved in with us about a month before our wedding. When we last saw the oncologist, she suggested we might want to move our wedding date up so that my mother could enjoy the festivities with us. It was her way of telling me that my mother might not make it until our wedding day. Gene and I discussed it, but everyone's airline tickets had been purchased, reception plans were made, and the like. So, I simply prayed that my mother would make it until our wedding, and she did.

Months earlier, when my mother was still healthy, she told me that she knew what she wanted to wear to my wedding. "I want to wear white sweater, pearls, and black slacks. Of course, when she originally envisioned this, she didn't know she was terminally ill, nor did I for that matter.

I spent a lot of the month of September planning our wedding. I always talked with my mom about the arrangements we were making. The kids would be there, her grandchildren, and many of our close friends and family. I talked about the flowers, the cake, the reception, and anything I could to keep her involved, including making her do chores. Every time I brought up a load of clean laundry from the basement, I brought it into her room.

"If you're going to live here, you've got to earn your keep," I always joked. Then I'd hand her washcloths and socks to fold. She'd roll her eyes if I put too much on her, but we laughed and had a good time.

Things were going quite well, but she was continuing to lose weight. She would eat a slice of toast here and an egg there, some pudding, and a protein drink occasionally, but for the most part she wasn't taking in enough calories to sustain her body. Try as we may, she ate less every day.

Her best friend, who had moved to Florida years earlier, came to visit her children in Connecticut in September. Dot had lost her husband to cancer two years earlier, and a daughter several months after that. She called to tell me she wanted to see my mother. I told her I would be at work, but Gene was home, so I told her to come and stay as long as she wanted.

She called me late in the day after her visit and said how shocked she was at my mother's condition. Before her visit in September, Dot had visited my mother at my home in July. Even then she mentioned that my mother was merely a shell of the person she knew. But when she saw her in September, she wasn't sure my mother would make it to my wedding, less than a month away. It was something I thought of many times.

Gene and I had decided to get married in our backyard and have our reception at a local Sicilian restaurant. We invited thirty-five guests, both friends and family. All the kids had a part in the wedding. Joe, my oldest, was the flower girl; Alex, my youngest, was the ring bearer; Emily, Gene's oldest, was the photographer; and Hannah, Gene's youngest, was the music director.

We hired a family friend to officiate the wedding, and asked Father Stan from Bishop Seabury Anglican Church to bless our union. I planned everything down to the last detail, most at one in the morning after I got home from work each day.

The Wedding

When I was married the first time, there was no such thing as the Internet. I lived in Florida and got married in Connecticut, so my parents planned and paid for everything. Even though I loved my first wedding, I was excited about planning this one.

Amazon became my late-night shopping Mecca. I could find almost everything there and have it shipped to arrive in two days. I bought a ten-foot-by-thirty-foot tent, an archway, a podium, invitations, the cake topper, and even my dress, from the comfort of my living room.

I asked my best friend, who was in my first wedding, to stand up for me this time around. She said she would if she got to pick the dress. My first wedding was the typical wedding—baby blue dresses that no one could wear again. I told her it was a deal. She picked out an elegant dark-blue dress that was knee length. It was perfect.

We also needed to get a suit for my father. He had walked me down the aisle the first time and was still here to walk me down the aisle again. It had been years since my dad had bought, or worn, a suit. Anything he had in his closet was five sizes too big, so we took him out to buy a new suit. We also had it professionally tailored. He looked so handsome. It was bittersweet, though, because I knew in the back of my mind that this was the suit that he would not only marry me in, but that I would bury him in—even if it was ten years from then.

At first, Gene struggled with who he wanted to stand up for him, but when we narrowed it down, the choice was obvious. In 2009, Gene got involved in a genealogy project. He has always been fascinated with his ancestry, so when he was approached to help with a project being sponsored by a local library, he jumped at the chance. It was during the project that he met Ed.

Gene and Ed became fast friends and worked on the project until 2015 when Ed died of multiple myeloma. Gene knew that if Ed had survived, he would have asked him to be his best man, but since he didn't, he asked his widow, Bonnie, to stand up with him. She accepted instantly.

We bought airline tickets and rented hotel rooms for the kids. We really wanted them to be there, so it was worth the cost to make sure that happened. We also made sure they had the correct outfits. Again, we wanted to make sure that whatever they were wearing they could use again, so we kept it simple: black pants and a black vest, and we would buy the cobalt-blue shirts to match Gene's.

I have always dreamed of having a kitchen big enough to hold a large farm table with enough seats to have huge dinners with family and friends. When we met with the owner of the Cantina, the local Sicilian restaurant in Middletown, he explained that he thought family style would be the best option. Since the party was small for a wedding, he thought that would be the most intimate, and since it had a table even longer than the one I had dreamed of, I thought it would be perfect.

I ordered my mother's sweater. It was beautiful, cream-colored, with pearls all along the neckline. I ordered her some simple black pants, some warm boots, and a beautiful cream-colored lap blanket. The wedding was going to be outside, so I wanted to make sure she was warm enough.

Finally, the day rolled around. It was a crisp October morning, but the weatherman said it would be in the seventies by late morning. Everything was decorated and ready for the wedding. I was so excited. I was in a hurry but managed to have a quick cup of coffee with my mother. I asked her if she felt up to the day, and she emphatically said yes.

We hired a private-duty nurse to be with my mom for the day. She would dress my mother for the wedding and then be with her at home while we were at the reception. She was far

The Wedding

too weak to attend the reception, but she was determined to be at the wedding.

After getting our hair done, Ann and I hunkered down at my neighbor's house next door. I could see people parking and coming into the yard. I watched as Gene and my sons maneuvered my mother's wheelchair out the front door and down the driveway to the backyard. Once she was in place, we asked that everyone take their seats.

As my father and I walked down the grass aisle towards the archway where Gene and Bonnie were standing, I looked around. Over the last months I had envisioned this scene over and over in my head. My future mother-in-law was on the right, near the front, across the aisle from my mother, who sat in her wheelchair wrapped in the lap blanket I bought her and wearing her sweater covered in pearls. It was exactly as I had envisioned it. I was overwhelmed with emotion.

I wanted the ceremony to be poignant, something that guests would remember as simple but meaningful. I decided that, along with the legal part, we needed a spiritual leader, and I wanted family members to read from the Bible.

Gene's sister, Elayne, read from Corinthians, and his nephew read from the Bible too. Dot read an essay she had written years earlier that had been published in a local newspaper at Christmastime:

> *God is love. I find that love in the smile of a child. I see it when I look at my spouse. I see it in my friends. It's there in the song of a bird and the wind in the trees. Love is in the wag of a dog's tail and purr of a cat. It's there in the smiles we give each other.*
>
> *This is the best time of year, the time for gifts. God's gift to us is love, and this is when we know it most. We do not earn*

it. It comes to every race, every creed and to all parts of the world. Our gift to others is to share that love.

We pass on God's love with every kind deed, with every smile, with every good thought.

Those smiles, those thoughts, are from God. When we turn away from bad deeds and thoughts, we use this gift.

This gift is ours, not just one day a year, but all year long.

Thank you, God.

I give you my smile.

Finally, Hannah, Gene's youngest daughter wrote and sang a song. The ceremony lasted just over fifteen minutes. It was perfect.

After the ceremony, Gene and the boys made sure my mother got back into the house safely. Even though she was only out of bed for twenty-five minutes or so, I could tell she was exhausted. After greeting all the guests, I made my way into the house to check on her. She was seated in her wheelchair in the living room, with my father seated on the couch beside her.

Just as I was walking in the front door, Father Stan was walking in the back. My mother-in-law had asked him to bring communion for my parents. He introduced himself to my parents and asked if he could pray over them. He asked God to watch over them, to stay close during this trying time, and to grant them peace and love. He gave them both communion and said a final blessing.

Once my mother was comfortably back in bed, we left for the reception. I kissed my mother on the forehead and told her I loved her and how happy I was that she was at my wedding. She nodded her head in agreement and whispered, "Me too."

We partied all weekend. All our children were in one place, which was rare, so we took full advantage of it and spent as much time together as we could. Gene and I set up a makeshift party room in the garage. This would allow us to spend time without being loud in the house, so my mother could rest. She took part in as much as she could, which consisted of being in the center of things in her wheelchair in the living room.

We had a dart board set up, plenty of chairs, and a table in the center where we set up a tame version of beer pong. The practical side of me thought that drinking beer from a glass that had a ping pong ball that had been bounced on the floor in it was not what I really wanted to do. So, we improvised and used water instead of beer. Don't get me wrong, we still managed to get our fair share of drinking in. Instead of drinking the beer that would normally have been in the red plastic cups, if we missed, we had to drink whatever was in *our* cup. A much better option.

We had a great time all weekend. The house was a mess, there were empty bottles everywhere, the yard was a wreck, but I was never happier.

Chapter Seven

The Unexpected

Depending on the time involved in your journey of caring for a sick person, there are many unexpected events that can arise that can throw a monkey wrench into the works. For me, it was a wedding and an automobile accident. The wedding I went over in the previous chapter. It was an amazing day, but bittersweet knowing that my mother was not going to be with us much longer. She was fading fast, only able to take in a couple hundred calories a day. She was trying to live, but the cancer was taking control, and she had little left to fight with.

In mid-October, I was running errands on my day off. I had a limited amount of time to shop for a pair of shoes for work and get back to the house before my mother's nurse arrived for his regular visit. There is an entrance ramp near my house that is well known for the number of accidents that occur there. Its location leaves no room for error. Traffic comes up over a hill at fifty-five miles per hour, and cars entering the highway do so from a complete stop. Not only does the person entering the highway have to be mindful of oncoming traffic, but the car next in line must be mindful of the car in front of them. Often, the first car in line does not move when others expect it to.

That was the case that morning. I was first in line to get onto the highway, and a car unexpectedly moved from the left lane, back into the right lane, obstructing my ability to merge onto the highway. The problem was that the car behind me was not looking at what I was doing and rammed into my back end. Keep in mind, I was on a time crunch. I pulled over and told the driver it was her lucky day; I didn't have time to wait for the police to show up. I took her information, asked her to call her insurance company, and went on my way.

Fast-forward almost a year later. The driver's insurance company paid for the damage to the car, which I had repaired, but they were less than gracious about paying my medical expenses. It had been over thirty years since I was involved in a car accident, so I was not aware of the games insurance companies now often played with claims. When all was said and done, the driver's insurance company offered me five hundred dollars less than my medical bills, which my doctor ended up writing off.

I did consult with a couple of attorneys, but since there was so little margin in the claim, they said they wouldn't take it on. Turns out that if I had "milked" the claim by calling out of work and requesting pain and suffering, I would have been able to sue them for five or six times what my medical expenses were. Just one more system that is corrupted.

Chapter Eight

The First Ending

After the wedding and everyone left, our house settled back into a routine. Gene and I were up early in the morning to change my mother and get her up for coffee. By mid-October, she was spending more time in bed sleeping, but she was still getting up twice a day for coffee. We could coerce her into eating once a day, but most of it was coming back up. Not only was she no longer able to swallow food, when she tried, she also brought up a lot of very thick mucus. It was so thick and sticky that she lost her breath as we pulled it out of her mouth.

I was working mostly closing shifts at this point. It allowed me time to get my mother ready for the day and spend some time with her in the morning when she was awake. I'd head to work by noon, and Gene would handle things from there.

On my days off, I tried to relieve Gene as much as possible, but often that meant I stayed with my mother while he took my father to the shore to tend to my parent's cat, who was living a sad, lonely existence in their old home.

My parents always had animals. When we were growing up, we always had a dog and at least one cat. In the last year, they had a dog that died and a 13-year-old cat that was still alive. When they moved in with us, we couldn't take their cat; we had three of our own. Therefore, we needed to plan to feed the cat and clean up after it. This went on from August until December.

The First Ending

Every two or three days, one of us drove to Old Lyme, cleaned up after the cat, and then gave her fresh food and water. She wasn't used to being inside all the time and had never used a cat box. She learned quickly but was not thrilled when it got dirty. Therefore, we had to place protective sheets all over the floor or she would pee right on it. The house smelled awful.

We emptied the litter, threw away the pads, and mopped the floor, all while feeding the cat can after can of food. We then put down multiple cans of food and dishes of dry food to tide her over, but she always seemed hungry when we got there, even though there was always dry food left in the bowl. We also got in the habit of letting her outside as soon as we got there.

It was a meager existence for a cat that was used to being spoiled every day, but I didn't have the heart to put her down, nor could I lie to my mother about how her cat was. Every time someone went to the shore to feed the cat, my mother would ask how she was.

One Wednesday after Gene and I finished grocery shopping, he decided to take my father to care for the cat. Taking my father added stress to the process, since he moved very slowly, but on this day we felt it would be good for him to get out of the house. He wasn't going out much, but then again, he didn't go out much before my mother's illness. I felt we needed to encourage it from time to time.

My mother was in the living room in her wheelchair having coffee when they decided to go. We contemplated whether to put her back in bed, but they were just going down and back, so she wouldn't be in the chair for more than an hour or so. She seemed perfectly comfortable, so we decided to leave her where she was. That was a huge mistake.

It was about five o'clock, so I poured myself a glass of wine and settled on the couch next to her. We sat quietly watching the news for about thirty minutes or so. What happened next, I wasn't clear about at the time, but suffice it to say it scared the crap out of me. Suddenly, my mother's head dropped down and her chin was resting on her chest. Then her head bobbed backwards, and her eyes opened wide.

I jumped up from where I sat on the couch and quickly got to her side. "Are you okay?" I asked. I could hear the nerves in my voice. "Mom, what's the matter?" She was staring at me blankly.

Then, as if nothing happened, she was fine. I could smell that she had soiled herself, but there wasn't anything I could do about it. I wasn't strong enough to get her to bed by myself. Then, once again, her head dropped and she started leaning in the chair. I held her up with the weight of my body pushing against hers. She was dead weight.

I grabbed my cell phone and started dialing. First, I called my neighbor to the left and asked if she was home. She was at her mother's house twenty minutes away. I hung up quickly and continued to dial. I dialed the hospice emergency line, and the nurse said she would have someone call back. My mother was still slumped over in the chair. Between calls, she gained consciousness and asked to go back to bed. I knew I couldn't get her into bed alone, so I called my other neighbor. I knew her mother was a nurse and she was visiting, so I was hoping she could come over. The call went to voicemail.

By this time, I was frantic. I was convinced that my mother was dying before my eyes and there was nothing I could do to help her. I called Gene. He was still forty minutes away but said he would get there as fast as he could. I told him to hurry, that my mother was having some type of seizures and they weren't stopping. His forty-minute trip turned out to be twenty-five, but it felt like a lifetime.

The First Ending

When he walked in the door, I was still standing by my mother's wheelchair, sweating from fear and having to hold her up. Gene quickly took over and got her into bed. We cleaned her up, got her some water, and settled her into bed. I breathed a sigh of relief and collapsed in his arms. I started to cry but pulled myself together quickly. I didn't want my father to see how scared I was.

That night we vowed that my mother would never be out of bed when Gene wasn't home. We found out that what happened was that she was having seizures or mini strokes. The nurse told us that now that she was no longer eating, her body lacked the vitamins and minerals she needed to stay alive. Her body was starting to shut down.

She had a couple more episodes like this, but Gene was there and could quickly get her back into bed. It only seemed to happen when she was sitting up in her wheelchair having coffee. By early November, she would have to sit on the edge of the bed to regain her balance before getting out of bed. We were patient with her and let her take whatever time she needed.

She was spending more time in bed watching TV and even more time sleeping. There were days when she didn't stir until later morning, then was back in bed by early afternoon. I no longer woke her to kiss her goodnight when I got home from work. I wanted her to rest.

On Thursday, November 10, I worked the closing shift. Gene texted me throughout the day with updates. Nothing unusual, but she didn't get out of bed to have coffee that day. He helped her with it in bed. At 6:30 that evening, he called me at work. "You better come home, hon," he said quietly. "She had another seizure, and I don't think she's coming out of this one. She's not responding."

I instantly called my boss, told him what was going on, and turned the store over to a key holder. I purposely drove home carefully, trying to stay in the moment. What I didn't want to do was get into an accident because I wasn't paying attention. I needed to get home quickly but safely.

When I walked in, my father was sitting on the couch watching TV. I greeted him, put my purse and lunchbox down, and went into my mother's bedroom. Gene was sitting in the pink chair by her bedside. He was holding her hand.

"How is she?" I whispered.

"She hasn't stirred," he said sadly. "It doesn't look good."

I went around the bed to the other side and put my hand in her hand. With the other hand, I pushed her hair back from her forehead. "Mom," I said a little loudly, "I'm here." Her eyes opened slightly, but only for a second, then she closed them again. Gene and I looked at each other, knowing this was the beginning of the end.

Neither my father nor Gene had eaten by that point, but I had finished dinner at work, so I told him I would sit with her while they ate something. We called the hospice number and told them what was happening. They said they would send the nurse out in the morning.

I sat with her for a long time that night. She was sleeping and didn't seem to be in any discomfort or pain, but she also wasn't responding. I asked my father if he wanted to sleep in another room that night, but he said no. He wanted to be there in case my mother needed him.

When I got up the next morning, my father was already coloring at the dining room table. "How's she doing?" I asked.

"She's fine, but she's snoring a lot," he said, chuckling.

When I checked in on her, I heard what he thought was snoring, but I knew better. What he was hearing was what they call the death rattle. When a person is in their final hours, the lungs begin to fill with liquid, making every breath crackle as the

The First Ending

lungs expand and contract. When I grabbed her hand to hold it, it was cold, but she was still breathing.

When Zack got there late the next morning, not much had changed. She was unconscious and unresponsive, and her breathing was labored now. We updated him on what happened the night before, and he made notes in his laptop.

"It sounds like she's actively dying," he explained. "Let me go check on her."

We waited a few minutes. When he came through the kitchen into the living room, I could tell by the look on his face that it wasn't good news.

"She's in duress," he said sadly. "She's breathing on top of her breathing, which is very painful." He went on. "We should really start giving her morphine. In most cases, it allows the patient to relax and the breathing will get easier. It won't be long though. She may be gone before the end of the day."

What I loved most about hospice is that they always took the time needed to make sure everyone involved was okay. After Zack gave us directions on how to administer the morphine, he went back into her room and moved her to make sure she was as comfortable as she could be. Then he sat with my father.

"Elizabeth isn't doing very well, Tony," he said in a gentle, soothing voice. "It looks like we're nearing the end. Are you okay?" My father said he was, and they chatted for a few more minutes.

As I said earlier, years ago when my father was ill, an operation and weeks of chemo and radiation treatments had saved his life. He didn't understand why the same couldn't happen for my mother. He had been frustrated with the rollercoaster ride we were taken on until the point that my mother was diagnosed with cancer. Once we got the diagnosis, he didn't understand why they couldn't operate and fix it. Although we tried to explain it, he just sucked his teeth in resignation and got angry.

Zack left my father in the dining room and rejoined Gene and me in the living room. "Have you made any arrangements for after she passes?" he asked. I told him I hadn't.

Once again, hospice came through, and Jan called me with several options. She explained that I should call each of them and, once I decided, I should let them know that my mother was hours away from dying.

I planned on going to work that day—distractions were a must for me those days—but Gene and my boss convinced me I needed to stay home to be there for my mom. Gene knew that sitting there waiting for my mother to die would drive me crazy, so he did what every good husband should do in those circumstances—he sent me shopping.

Gene handed me a grocery list and shooed me out the door. As I look back, we probably didn't need half of what was on that list, but he knew it was what I needed, something to keep me busy.

I wandered around the grocery store for hours. Perhaps my subconscious mind thought that if I stayed there I wouldn't have to face what was happening in the real world, that somehow the safety of that grocery store would prolong my mother's life, but my conscious mind knew that would never happen. Part of the reason that I moved back to Connecticut was soon going to end. It left my heart heavy.

When I got home, Gene helped me with the groceries. Because I spent so much time in the store, I bought far more than we needed, but I justified it by knowing that none of it would go to waste. I checked on my mom; she seemed to be breathing easier. I did notice her breathing had slowed considerably, but it was no longer crackling. I checked on my father too, who

The First Ending

seemed to be doing well under the circumstances. While I know he was aware of what was going on, he seemed unaffected by it. He had a funny way of dealing with life—and death, for that matter.

I spent a lot of time holding my mother's hand that day. It was cold, stiff, and unresponsive, but I still held on. I wanted her to know that she wasn't alone, that I was keeping my promise to be with her till the end, that we were a team.

By 10:30 that night, I was falling asleep in the chair beside her. We had been administering morphine all day, so I knew she wouldn't last much longer. I silently said my goodbye, kissed her good night, and went to bed. I knew it would be the last time I saw her alive.

As I turned to leave, I thought back to a conversation we had on Tuesday of that week. Her room was dark, and I was getting her ready for bed. "Aren't you tired of this?" she asked yet again.

I responded the same way I did every time she asked that question. "I would do this for the rest of my life, if given the chance." She always smiled at that. Once I tucked her in, I settled in the pink chair next to her bed. She shut the TV off and turned towards where I was sitting.

"Do you think it's time to say goodbye?" she asked.

My eyes welled up instantly. "I'm not ready," I said through my tears. "Are you?"

She shook her head from side to side. I smiled. We sat there silently, both lost in our own thoughts.

"I will tell you this though," I said, my voice quivering. "One of these days we're going to decide to meet on the other side." She pointed her finger up in agreement.

"Go get some rest; it's late," she said, not realizing it was only 5:30 in the afternoon, but I kissed her and turned her light off.

"I love you, Elizabeth," I said.
"Love you too," she said right back.

***

When I left her bed that last night, I told her that we would all be okay. I thanked her for giving me the opportunity to care for her. I thanked her for finally being the mother I always needed her to be. I told her I loved her and that it was okay to let go. And lastly, I told her I'd meet her on the other side. Then I turned and walked out, never looking back.

Gene and I woke very early the next morning and laid in the bed for a few minutes. "What time did you come to bed?" I asked.

"I gave her a dose of morphine at 12:30 and came to bed. You were snoring when I got in," he explained.

I was usually snoring when he came to bed. I have always had an uncanny knack of falling asleep quickly. Gene has always commented on it. I think he's just jealous.

It was 5:30 in the morning when we made our way downstairs to check on my mother. I lagged behind while Gene looked in on her. He came back to the living room seconds later and told me she was gone. I walked behind him into the room. My father was still asleep in his bed, so I softly nudged him. When he stirred, I told him that she was gone.

"I know," he said. My first thought was that he had sensed it during the night, but his next statement corrected that. "I got up to pee about 2:30 and she was gone," he said matter-of-factly.

I was shocked. "Why didn't you wake us?"

"I don't know," he replied. Thinking back, it may have been the time he needed to say goodbye.

I helped him get out of bed and took him into the living room. I then called the hospice line to let them know she had

The First Ending

died. They gave their condolences and said they would send someone out to declare her within the hour.

Gene made coffee and we waited for the nurse to arrive. My father was very quiet but said he was okay. It was still very early in the morning, so calling anyone to let them know what happened was out of the question. When 6:30 rolled around, Dad asked me to call his sister.

Paula was a huge support system throughout my mother's illness. She called every day for an update and to see how we were all doing. She lived too far away to visit, but her calls were often a release for me, someone I could talk to.

When I told her the news, she started crying immediately. Paula has always been a crier. It's her way of releasing, so I let her cry. She asked a few questions about the arrangements, none of which I was prepared to answer, so I told her I would call later in the day once things were rolling.

Once the nurse arrived, she listened to my mother's heart, cleaned her up, and wrote the time on her death certificate. She was declared dead at 7:43 a.m. The nurse then called the funeral home and asked them to come pick up the body. She said it would be an hour or so before they could get there, which wasn't a problem; it wasn't like she was going anywhere.

The van from the funeral home pulled up in front of the house at 8:30. Two young men knocked on the door. When I opened it, they both offered their condolences. I showed them where my mother's room was, asked them if they needed anything, and told them I was going to bring my father upstairs. None of us wanted to see her being removed from the house.

Gene and I helped my father upstairs and got him situated in a chair. I knew it was time to call my brother and sister. They had been estranged from my mother and father for years, but I felt it was the right thing to call them and let them know that Mom had passed away.

I pulled up the last number I had for my brother and hit send on my cell phone. I got a message that the number was disconnected and no longer in service. Recently, I had reconnected with my brother's ex-wife, so I called her through Facebook. She picked up right away. I told her that Mom had passed away earlier that morning and that I needed my brother's phone number. She gave it to me, we chatted briefly, I told her to give the kids my love, and I hung up.

When I dialed the number she'd given me, my brother picked up on the second ring. "I have some bad news," I said. My brother and I hadn't spoken in years. He and my mother didn't get along. They never seemed to get past everything that happened when he was young; he had been quite a hellion. "Mom passed away this morning."

"Wow," was his response. Then there was silence.

"She's had cancer for the last year." Again, silence. "Look, I just thought you should know," I said and hung up the phone.

Then I called my sister. She didn't answer. My first thought was that she was nursing a hangover and it was too early, but I left a message anyway. "Hey there, it's Barb. Give me a call when you get this message."

I hung up the phone, thinking she would call within the hour, but that wasn't the case. In fact, I called again around noon and she still didn't answer the phone. She finally picked up when I called back around five o'clock.

She sounded groggy when she answered the phone. "Hello?" she said. Her voice was raspy, but I was used to that. Years of smoking and drinking will do that to a person.

"Listen, I have some bad news," I said quietly into the phone.

The First Ending

She started crying instantly and screaming into the phone. "Noooo." She screamed without even knowing what the news was.

I waited for her to settle down.

"Mom passed away this morning," I said and waited for her response.

Hers was completely different than my brothers. Instead of saying nothing or reacting like my brother had, she started yelling at me. "Why didn't you say that on the answering machine?"

I was dumbfounded. "I didn't think you would want to hear that your mother died on a voicemail message," I said, not believing that I was having to justify my actions.

"I didn't even know she was sick!" she continued to yell.

"She didn't want you to know," I said.

It was true. Only once during her illness had my mother mentioned my brother or sister. It was only in the context of her wondering what they would think of her being sick. When I asked if she wanted me to call them, she said no. She believed that if they didn't want to be part of her life, then they didn't deserve to be part of her death. I told my sister that, which she didn't like. She continued yelling at me and I stopped her. I had finally had enough.

"Look, I don't know who you think you are yelling at me. I simply called to let you know that Mom died. I don't have to listen to you yell at me anymore. Goodbye." And I hung up the phone. I thought the whole thing was surreal. My mother had died that morning, my brother was indifferent, and my sister was a screaming maniac. Some things never changed.

My father asked about each of the conversations, and I was honest with him. I wanted to make sure he wasn't delusional about his other children. He never understood why my brother and sister had distanced themselves from him and my mother.

It bothered him and made him worry, but as the years went by, his worry turned to anger. He often said he might never forgive them.

Over the years, my mother had a habit of stopping my father whenever the subject of my brother and sister was brought up. That day, however, she wasn't there to stop him, and I let him go. I thought it would be a way for him to purge his emotions, to let it all go. And I was right, once he got it all out—the pain, the disappointment, the anger, and frustration—he handled the whole situation much better. When he was done, I took his hands and we prayed for both of them. We asked God to stay near them, guide them closer to him, and keep them safe. My father was clear that he didn't want to speak of them again.

The day after my mother died, I thought it was important that we all get out of the house. Gene and my father had been trapped by my mother's illness, and the only time I was out of the house was to work. So, we decided to go down to the shore, feed the cat, check on the house, and then go to dinner with Paula. I asked my father where he wanted to go for dinner, knowing he would want to go to Olive Garden.

For the last four or five years, my mother hadn't cooked much, maybe an occasional meal when we visited, which was usually overcooked and dried out. Since she wasn't cooking, most nights he was left to fend for himself while she ate some frozen something out of a box. Even though my father was Italian, he didn't know how to cook much. He was an expert at cooking pasta out of a box, though, so that's what he ate most of the time, but he loved the eggplant at Olive Garden, so he always wanted to go there when we went out.

While we were waiting to be seated at the restaurant, I checked my phone to make sure I hadn't missed any calls. I hadn't, but I saw there was a text message from my brother. I won't go

The First Ending

into all the details, but I will say that it was extremely nasty. He said horrible things about my mother, that she was a bitch and that she had kept my brother from having a relationship with my father for years. He went on to say that he wanted to talk to our father and that I should facilitate that happening, unless I planned on perpetuating the angst that my mother created. He went on to say how he and my sister were the black sheep of the family, that I was always the favored one, and that we were all tortured as children.

I'll admit that our upbringing was not an episode from the *Brady Bunch*, but I didn't recall being tortured. My mother and my brother were at odds most of the time. He was difficult, and she was tired of his antics. He is five years older than me, so much of it I don't remember.

My sister joined the Army shortly after we graduated. I was never close to her while we were growing up. She was lazy, and I had to pick up a lot of the slack, which didn't lend itself to us being close. She was a bit of a drama queen—another thing I had little tolerance for—but she had learned that she got attention when she was dramatic, so it worked for her. She had separated herself from the family ten years earlier when she met her most recent boyfriend, John. She had a habit of bringing us into her life only when it was falling apart. It was sad but true.

At dinner, I showed the text messages to Gene. Before I handed him my phone, I whispered in his ear that he shouldn't react when he read them. I wanted to protect my father. He had been through enough. After Gene read it, he couldn't help but be angry at the words, but he kept it together.

On the ride home, I sat in the back seat with my father. We had to talk. As much as I didn't like the way my brother and sister had treated my parents, I couldn't keep them apart if my father wanted them in his life. I had to let him know about the messages my brother sent and let him decide how he wanted to handle it.

The one thing I swore I wouldn't do is welcome my brother or sister into my home. After how they treated my parents, their reaction to my mother's death, and my brother's harsh words, I vowed I would not allow them back into my life. They were far too caustic.

As Gene drove, I gave my father a watered-down version of what my brother said. I did let him know that my brother felt he was tortured as a child and that he felt like my mother had kept them apart for years. This made my father angry, which I didn't expect.

"Your brother was the one who chose to distance himself. After he left the Navy, everything changed. He never took my advice or listened to what I had to say." He was getting all worked up. He even dropped a couple of F-bombs—something he never did.

I went on to tell him that my brother wanted to see him or talk to him. Dad had no interest in either. "When he gets sober and gets things right with God, I'll think about it." And that was the end of the conversation.

My father had spent the last year watching his wife die. It had taken a toll on him emotionally and physically. My main concern after my mother died was to care for him and make sure he would be okay.

My sister and brother thought otherwise. My brother continued to call my parent's phone at their old house, only to leave messages about how much he missed his "Poppy." At first, I told my father about the messages. Then, when I saw how angry it made him, I stopped. I also disconnected the answering machine.

My sister took things to a whole new level. She began calling my Aunt Paula and leaving threatening messages on her

The First Ending

answering machine. At one point, she left a message threatening to contact an attorney if she was not allowed to speak to her father, as if not speaking to someone was a criminal offense. I cautioned my aunt not to pick up calls from her number, and then I got my father involved.

My father was quite angry when he heard that his daughter was threatening his sister. He decided it was time to intervene. "If she wants to talk to me, then I'll call her. Enough is enough," he said.

I was on my way to work, so I gave Gene my sister's phone number and left. When he and my father called, they got her voicemail.

My father left a very brief message. "This is your father. I've heard that you want to talk to me. I need you to call me before the end of the day today. Goodbye." He handed Gene his cell phone and shook his head.

Several hours later Gene's phone rang; it was my sister. He answered and asked her to hang on while he handed the phone to my father, who was sitting in the dining room coloring. Gene handed him the phone and left him alone. He didn't want to be part of the conversation.

We don't live in a large house, so trying not to listen to my father's end of the conversation wasn't easy. From the living room, Gene could hear clearly what my father was saying, and it wasn't good. He recounted that the gist of the conversation was that she needed to get her "shit together," stop drinking, and get things right with God, that he didn't want anything to do with her until she had done this, and that she needed to stop calling and harassing his sister. Then he hung up the phone.

***

But it wasn't the end of the harassment. My brother continued to send me text messages that were rude and condescending. Most of them I ignored, but it finally got to a point where I could no longer take it. One afternoon I was off from work and he started again. His messages usually came in after five and were rambling and confusing to read. I knew he was drinking, just by the tone of his messages. This day I had enough. I called him.

The conversation lasted about twenty minutes. There was a lot of screaming and yelling and swearing. I told him he had no idea what we had been through in the last year, that Dad was old and feeble and didn't need, or want, any drama in his life. I also told him that Dad didn't want to speak to him and that I didn't want him in my life. My brother had a habit of calling me "baby sister," with a condescending tone that let me know he thought he was more important than I was. I told him I would pray for him every day and hope that God remained close to him. Then I told him to leave me alone, hung up the phone, and blocked his number.

Chapter Nine

A New Beginning

After my mother died, my father toyed with the idea of living alone in their house in Old Lyme. Gene and I were concerned about this for a couple of reasons. The first was that he had fallen twice in the last few months. He was very unstable on his feet and lost his balance easily. Being thirty minutes away would drive me crazy, thinking he had fallen and was not able to get up. The second was the fact that I didn't think he would do well living alone. I was afraid that he would sit in the house alone and wither away. He had never lived alone in his entire life, and I didn't think he would like it.

After several discussions, we decided that he would live with us through the winter and we would revisit the idea come spring. He seemed resigned to the fact, but once he thought about it, he knew it was for the best.

So, we settled into a new routine. Dad helped with chores around the house, took care of himself and his room, and integrated himself into our routines. It was working quite well. He seemed happy with the arrangement, but he was concerned because he thought he should miss my mother more. I told him not to worry about it. She had been difficult the last several years, so it only made sense that he didn't miss that, but I know it bothered him.

The holidays were right around the corner, and I was concerned how my father would handle the first of many firsts without my mother—first Thanksgiving, first Christmas, etc. When I talked to him about what he wanted to do, he said he wanted things the way they had always been. He was a creature of habit and a man of tradition. It all made perfect sense.

On Thanksgiving morning, I went to pick up my aunt, and Gene stayed behind to get the turkey ready. My father stayed with him to help. We had all the fixings, even the corn pudding my mother loved. At the beginning of the meal, we toasted my mother and all the other family members no longer with us. It was a wonderful day.

Christmas was much of the same—although my father did his Christmas shopping online for the first time in his life, with Gene's help of course. He wasn't much for getting out in the cold weather, so he stayed home most of the time, even when Gene and I invited him out with us.

My father was living on one floor in our home—his bedroom and bathroom were on the first floor—but Gene and I were always concerned for his safety. We wanted to replace the existing tub with a walk-in shower. In January, we hired a contractor, my hairdresser's husband, to help us renovate his bathroom. The commotion from the construction seemed to be good for my dad. He was always interested in watching someone build things. He wasn't very handy himself, but he loved to watch and put in his two cents.

The winter months were uneventful. I found a new doctor for my father, a practice that specialized in geriatric medicine. His new doctor was a young man who was on an internship for four years while working towards his residency. At our first visit, I voiced my concerns about my father being on so many different medications.

In the previous five years, my father had become obsessed with his weight. He was 120 pounds soaking wet. Try as he might, he never gained any weight. Several years earlier, I had put together a chart with all the probable and possible side effects from his medications. It was alarming to find out that some of them caused high blood pressure, which he was also being treated for. Others could cause false readings on things such as blood sugar tests; he was being treated for type-two diabetes. Others caused unexplained weight loss or the inability to keep weight on.

When I spoke with his new doctor, he suggested we leave things as they were to get a baseline, then adjust things one at a time so we could monitor the results. He did suggest that we get my father to a podiatrist.

Years earlier, veins had been taken from my father's legs and used for his heart. This left him with poor circulation in his legs, and his feet suffered. He had ulcers on his toes and under his toenails. His previous doctor had never even looked at his feet. In fact, my father said his doctor visits were the same every time—the nurse took his weight and blood pressure, the doctor listened to his heart and lungs, asked him how he was feeling, end of visit.

Now, in slight defense, my parents never told their doctor about any concerns, unless it was so blaring that they couldn't avoid it. I always felt their doctor was more concerned about handing them a prescription for whatever symptom they had than addressing the reason for the symptom. I also felt my parents' health was compromised by their own doing, from a poor diet, lack of exercise, and lack of interaction with other people. My father had long given up working in the yard, which had been his only form of exercise before his most recent heart attack.

My mother thought it was a great idea to get a dog for my father to walk. In theory, it was a good idea, but the dog she chose turned out to be a basket case. She was a white Shih Tzu named Sophie. When my mother saw her at the Humane Society, I warned her that she would be high maintenance, the kind of dog that required regular bathing and grooming. However, against my better judgement, she took Sophie home.

Sophie was rescued off the streets of Hartford. Life on the streets had left her hard and tainted against humans. I could only guess that she was neglected, at the very least. It only took a matter of days before she bit my father the first time. I was infuriated.

"She's gotta go," I said while I examined the dog bite on my father's arm.

"She's fine," my mother said, defending the dog's actions. "Your father just reached for her too quickly."

I rolled my eyes in disgust. This began two years of my father having to take care of this crazy dog who growled at him and bit him. It was a complete disaster. The vet bills were ridiculous; Sophie had bad eye and ear infections the entire time my parents owned her. She also wouldn't let my parents bathe her, so she went to the groomer every three weeks, until Sophie bit the groomer and they would no longer take her.

Finally, Sophie died. She had some intestinal issues that my parents were treating her for, and my mother found her dead on the kitchen floor one morning. It was a blessing in disguise.

***

By spring, things changed with my father. He was no longer changing his clothes or participating much in chores around the house. He would get up early in the morning, take a nap for several hours, watch TV, eat dinner, and go back to bed. I'd asked him if he wanted to do anything. We had a new community

A New Beginning

center within walking distance of our house. I thought maybe he would like to get involved in something there, but he didn't. He was perfectly happy with his routine.

In late March, Dad came down with a cold. It was just a common cold, the kind that goes away in seven days, but it scared him. He wanted to take all kinds of medication to mask the symptoms. His body didn't react well to any of them. One evening, about three days into his cold, he told Gene he wasn't feeling well. His chest hurt, and he was having a hard time breathing. Gene called me at work to let me know he was taking my father to the hospital.

After their initial exam, the doctors determined my father had pneumonia. The reason he was having such a hard time breathing was that his left lung was filling up with fluid. They admitted him and put him on Lasix to clear the lung and antibiotics to clear the pneumonia. He was there for four days, hating every minute of it.

With both my parents, I was always frustrated with their impatience in the hospital. Instead of doing something to prevent going there in the first place, like taking an active role in their own health, they did nothing and wound up in the hospital, complaining the whole time. I was always concerned that their agitation aggravated whatever was going on, because they didn't allow their bodies to relax and heal.

Because of the fluid in my father's lungs, the doctors talked about sending him home on oxygen. He was not able to keep his blood oxygen level where it needed to be, but towards the end of his stay, he could maintain it well enough. So, they sent him home without it.

My father didn't like being old. He didn't like the way he looked, often commenting about his skin hanging off his body. I reminded him that being old was better than the alternative, being dead, but I don't think he was ever really convinced. In his world, being fat was being healthy, and he was anything but fat.

He obsessed about his cancer coming back. Even though it hadn't returned in over twenty-five years, he was convinced that the reason he was so thin was because of cancer. Keep in mind that he had just watched my mother wither away in less than a year, so to him it made sense.

He was also afraid of dying. Now, mind you, every one of us has some fear of dying and going into the unknown, but I often said that my father had an unhealthy fear of it. He thought about it and talked about it far too often. This conversation would always go the same way. He would tell me or Gene that he was afraid of dying. We would tell him that none of us knew when it would be our time, and that it was in God's hands. We would also remind him that his faith taught him that once God was done with us on earth, he would take us home to be with him in heaven. I got the sense that he could never quite grasp that concept.

It got to the point that I spoke to his doctor about it and consulted with friends and family. Then I decided I would have to help him ease his fears. So, the next time he brought up his fear of dying, I told him each time he felt afraid that I wanted him to pray. I told him to ask God to help him with his fear and to comfort him. I don't think it ever really worked.

***

In May, my youngest son confirmed that he and his fiancée would be getting married in July. Although they both lived in Florida, she was originally from North Carolina, so they were going to have the ceremony there. Gene and I planned on renting a house for several days, with plenty of room for my father if he wanted to go.

A New Beginning

When I broached the idea of travelling with us to him, he wasn't thrilled about the idea. Even though fully recuperated from the pneumonia, it had taken a toll on him. He was no longer interested in coloring, didn't change his clothes, and was showering less. I had to talk to him several times about showering at least once a week and changing his clothes on a regular basis.

A day or so after I brought up my son's wedding, Dad told me he didn't want to go. Honestly, I was a little relieved. I knew the fourteen-hour drive, which we still did in one day, would be very hard on him. Then, all the activity surrounding the wedding would be exhausting.

We decided to have Gene's youngest daughter stay at the house with Dad while we were gone. She was working locally, so it would work out perfectly. She was working third shift, so we also asked our neighbor to check in on him during the day. We made his favorite meals in advance. By this time, he was eating a very limited diet, by his own choice. His favorites were macaroni and cheese and egg custard.

Shortly after my parents moved in with us, we made it clear that they could have whatever they wanted to eat. I felt that at this point, with my mother dying and my father underweight, that I would be hard pressed to correct any damage done by their poor diet.

My father's first request was egg custard. Over the years, I had tasted my father's rendition of egg custard, which ranged from a soupy mess to sweet scrambled eggs. By the time we left for North Carolina, Gene had become an expert at making it. It was a weekly ritual for him to whip up a batch. Two days before we left, he made a double batch. We made macaroni and cheese for him, also a double batch. We also packed in some apple turnovers, his morning staple with coffee. All this would tide him over for the four days we would be gone. It would only require a heat up in the microwave.

I explained to my dad when we would be leaving, who would be coming to check on him and when, and when we would be returning.

We left early on the fourth of July. The wedding was on Friday the seventh, so we decided that travelling on the fourth made sense, no one else would be on the road. We were right; the trip was smooth sailing. We made the fourteen-hour trip in twelve hours. It was nice to be away, but I was still anxious about leaving my father at home.

The wedding went off without a hitch. My youngest son was married to his beautiful bride, and it was time to go home. We left the morning of the eighth. This would give me a day at home before I had to return to work. It was a longer trip going home; we finally arrived at one in the morning. My dad was sound asleep.

When we got up the next morning, my father was there to greet us. We caught him up on the happenings during our trip, and he caught us up on his week. He said he had a good week but was glad we were home. We quickly settled back in.

Late in the day, I noticed that Dad kept looking from his wristwatch to the clock that hung on the wall in the kitchen. At first, I didn't think much of it, but then I noticed he was checking every few minutes.

"Dad, what are you doing?" I asked.

"I'm trying to match the time here to the time on the wall." He pointed to his wristwatch. I thought maybe the battery in his watch was dying, but the time was the same. I told him to relax and started to make dinner. He ate well that night and went to bed early.

The next day I went to work. Gene texted me to tell me that my father was once again matching his watch to the clock on the wall. He said he was doing it continuously at some points but then would relax for a while. I chalked it up to him worrying about us while we were gone, not really knowing when we were coming home.

Tuesday, I was off from work. I was busy running errands, so I hadn't spent much time with Dad during that day. When I got home, he was sitting on the couch. He was looking from his watch to the clock but wasn't saying anything. Then he started taking things off the table near where he sat. He was holding several lottery tickets I'd bought him for Father's Day. He hadn't scratched them off yet.

He laid each of the cards on the tray table in front of him and looked at each of them, puzzled.

"Dad, what are you doing?" I asked.

"I'm trying to match them up. Do these match?" he asked, holding two of the cards up.

I quickly learned that his matching had no rhyme or reason to it. It didn't have to do with the color of the cards, or the shape, or anything for that matter. I also realized that if I didn't help him match up the cards that he wasn't going to relax, so I played along. As soon as he matched two cards, I would agree that they matched and take them away. This continued until everything on his table was matched and had been taken away from him—hearing aids, glasses, cards. Once it was all gone from his sight, he relaxed.

After he went to bed, Gene and I talked about what happened. We both agreed that he was exhibiting signs of dementia and that this might be the new normal for him. We agreed that we would no longer be able to leave him by himself, which meant whatever small amount of freedom Gene had was completely gone. He was stuck in the house with my dad, except on my days off.

On Wednesday, I went to work. I was closing that day. Around 6:30, Gene called me to tell me that my father wasn't doing well. He was having a hard time breathing and wanted to go to the hospital. He told Gene he didn't feel strong enough to walk, so Gene called an ambulance. He kept me updated throughout the night by text message. When I finally left work at midnight, Gene was still in the emergency room.

Gene told the doctors about the matching and the new level of confusion we were seeing in the last couple of days. They didn't think much about it. Preliminary tests showed that my father had extremely low sodium levels in his body. The doctors were alarmed by this more than anything. My father's doctor had recently changed one of his medications. One of the side effects was a sudden drop in sodium levels, which could cause confusion and result in strokes, heart attacks, or death.

This, coupled with the fact that my father was very dehydrated, led to him being admitted. We had told my father that he never drank enough liquids. His doctor agreed. My father's daily consumption of fluids was usually a cup of coffee in the morning, Diet Pepsi with lunch, and a blackberry brandy and Pepsi concoction he mixed up with dinner.

Gene called him the Mix Master. My father had a weird habit of premixing brandy and Pepsi in bottles. He'd pour a small amount of blackberry brandy into an empty bottle and fill it the rest of the way with Pepsi. He said he didn't like the fizz in the Pepsi, so this way it would go flat before he drank it. I thought it was gross, but to each his own.

"We think your father had a heart attack," a doctor from the hospital explained to me the next morning.

By now they had my father on an IV of saline solution and some other medications to get his sodium levels up. They also

A New Beginning

had him on a very restricted diet. They restricted his salt intake, which I thought to be funny since his sodium levels were low.

After five days, they released him from the hospital. This time they sent him home with oxygen. While he was at rest, he could maintain a healthy blood oxygen level, but as soon as he got up to do something, it plummeted to the eighties. The doctors were concerned. When they released him, the discharging nurse said they would have a visiting nurse come to the house in the morning to check on him.

My father was so happy to be going home. Remember, we lived only a mile from the hospital, so we didn't think it would be a big deal getting him home and comfortable, but by the time we got him into the house, we were once again concerned. He had a really hard time getting from the car to the house on his own, so Gene helped him. He almost had to push my dad into the house because he was having such a hard time climbing the two steps in.

Once we got him in the house and settled, it dawned on me that we hadn't put his oxygen on when we left the hospital. We quickly turned on the machine the medical supply company had delivered to our home and put the tube in his nose. As he sat there breathing in the oxygen, he seemed to be relaxing. When I look back, I am convinced that my father had a stroke during the ride home. He wasn't feeling well and had a greyish color about him.

The nurses came late the next morning. I was getting ready for work while they were still examining my father. Gene called me while I was driving.

"They don't think it's safe for him to be here. The nurse doesn't think they should have released him. She's calling his doctor now."

As we hung up, I told him to keep me posted. Five minutes later, he texted me and said they were taking my dad to the hospital by ambulance. I knew my dad would be mad that he had to go back, but I also knew it was for the best.

Chapter Ten

A Turn for the Worse

In the back of my mind, I knew that this was the beginning of the end for my father. His health was failing quickly, and so was his mind. I wasn't sure what was happening, and neither did the doctors. When he ended up back at the hospital under the recommendation of the nurses who checked in on him, you can imagine my surprise when I got a call from his primary care physician at four o'clock that afternoon telling me that they were releasing my dad from the emergency room.

"Wait a minute," I said. "It hasn't even been six hours since your nurses called an ambulance to get my father back to the hospital, and you're going to release him? That's crazy."

The doctor went on to tell me that the tests still showed that his sodium levels were low, but they were on the rise, and he felt confident that trend would continue.

I interrupted him. "Doctor, something happened between yesterday and today. My father is very confused, sometimes incoherent. Something is going on. I don't want you to release him prematurely, just to turn around to admit him again tomorrow. Each time we do this, it takes a toll on him. Let's step back a bit and at least observe him overnight. If he's okay tomorrow, we'll talk about the options."

He wasn't buying it.

"Look, I'm on my way to the hospital; let me get there and see how he's doing."

I hung up the phone, frustrated. I took a couple of deep breaths and continued my drive home. I knew that if I let this get the best of me, the only one who would suffer was my father.

When I got to the hospital and walked into his room in the ER, I knew he wasn't leaving the hospital that day. He knew who I was and said hello, but something was very wrong. His hands were twisted in a weird position, and he kept raising his arms in the air. It was as if he had no control over his movements. Gene and I looked at each other. At that moment, a female doctor came into the room.

She introduced herself and said she called the doctor who released my father the day before. She wanted his opinion on my father's condition. She too—although she did not know what—believed something happened between the day before and today.

We waited for the doctor while my father rested. When he entered the room, the doctor introduced himself and addressed my father. It took him only a few minutes to realize something happened. The doctor had my father do some fine motor skill exercises, which he failed miserably. He couldn't touch his finger to his nose, even with his eyes open.

"Well, this certainly isn't the same man I discharged yesterday," he said. "I'm not sure what happened, but I think it would be wise to keep him overnight for observation."

Finally, someone was making some sense! After they admitted him and he was resting in his room, Gene and I went home.

The next morning, I got a call from his primary doctor. He was clear that my father was in no medical danger. He also agreed that something was going on, but he wasn't sure what. He said it may be a combination of heart attacks and strokes, but without extensive testing, they wouldn't know for sure. He went on to say that even with testing, which would be hard on him, there was nothing they could do. He was not a candidate for any kind of surgery in his compromised state.

The doctor recommended we consider a rehab center for a couple of weeks to get him stronger. He had been in a hospital bed for much of the last three weeks, so he was much weaker. He could barely walk on his own. He was using a walker, but still needed help to get to the bathroom and bed. His doctor thought with regular physical therapy and round-the-clock medical monitoring, that my father would get stronger and it would be safer for him to come home. I knew he would be upset, but I also knew it was for the best.

For the next ten days, my dad was in a rehab center. The place was one hundred times better than the one my mother had been in. It didn't smell, was nicely decorated, and the staff seemed more attentive. I was relieved, knowing that he was well taken care of.

My father was still very confused and had little control over his movements. This meant Gene or I would have to go to the center twice a day to make sure he ate. The rehab center could have an aide do it, but we knew he likely wouldn't cooperate with them. He was so mad at me for putting him there that he was punishing me by not eating, and he started talking about things that made no sense. It started the first time Gene went to give him lunch.

"He wanted me to take everything off the table," Gene told me when he called me after feeding him lunch. "Even the placemats were making him mad."

This was all new territory for us. My mother had all her faculties right up to the point when she slipped into a coma two days before her death. So, the mental confusion was new for us, and we didn't know how to handle it.

A Turn for the Worse

He would ask us to take him out of the room, or take everything out of the room, or take him out of this place. It was all too much. His eating habits changed as well. He started wolfing down food, barely taking time to breathe. We told him he had to eat to get stronger, but we were careful not to talk about going home, because we now weren't sure it would happen.

For the most part he was cooperative with the staff. They grew to love him quickly and looked after him. He kept to himself, but the staff was concerned about him being alone. He kept trying to get up by himself, take his oxygen tube out, or even take his clothes off. There were many times we would find him sitting in the hallway near the nurse's station when we arrived because they wanted to keep an eye on him.

He also was not sleeping at night. The nurses said he would sleep for a few hours and then want to get up. It could have been that his days and nights were confused, but more likely he was afraid to sleep for fear he would never wake up.

As the days went on, he became more and more agitated being in the rehab center. I talked with the doctor about bringing him home and continuing physical therapy at home. Medicare would cover it, along with a nurse, if they felt there was a medical need. So, we prepared to bring him home. The funny thing is, as soon as we gave my father the actual day we were going to bring him home, he stopped asking us to clear the room, take the placemats off the table, etc.

Chapter Eleven

Our Overnight Angel

Once we brought my father home, it was a completely different experience from when we brought my mother back from the rehab center. My mother had all her faculties about her and was very willing to play by the rules—meaning she was never to try to get out of bed on her own. She had a call button that she could use if she needed us during the night, but she rarely used it. Without us knowing it, she was the easier of the two to care for at night.

My father wasn't bedridden, nor was he on hospice care. Gene and I figured out a routine, but we were concerned about the nights. My father was a fall risk, totally confused, and very weak. He had to walk with a walker and was slow even at that.

By this time, his fear of dying in his sleep, along with other anxieties he mustered up in his mind, made sleep almost nonexistent. I was still working sixty to seventy hours a week, which left most of the burden on Gene. For him to be able to take care of my father during the day, we would need help at night.

There are hundreds of agencies claiming to offer services for overnight companionship. At the beginning, we thought it would be reasonable to hire someone to sit with my father for an eight-hour shift so Gene could get much-needed rest. It sounds simple, and we thought it wouldn't be too expensive—until you add in bodily functions. To hire someone capable of bringing my father to the bathroom during the night, the fee jumped from $150 a night to a minimum of $279. To have someone come in five nights a week, the bill would be a minimum of $1,400 per week, or over $5,000 per month, much more than my father's pension and Social Security could afford.

The woman who had been our housekeeper for the previous year had suddenly and tragically lost her fiancé. She told Gene she needed a new start, so she was going to start caring for the elderly. We were sad to see her go, but totally understood her need for a new beginning. So, when the thought of having someone come to be with my father during the night came up, I instantly thought of Kasia.

When I contacted her, she let me know that she already had a job, but her sister-in-law was looking for work. Even though I had never met Anna, I knew that Kasia was a good person and wouldn't steer me wrong. I'm not sure Anna had any formal training, except for CPR and first aid, but what she did have was a caring nature, a soft spot in her heart for the elderly, and hands-on experience.

I got Anna's phone number, and after a few text messages back and forth, we agreed on a hundred dollars a night; she was to start the very next day. While the two thousand dollars a month would exhaust my father's monthly income, at least it would be more manageable. We arranged that Anna would come at eleven o'clock each night and leave by six in the morning. Gene would stay up until she got there and then set his alarm so she could leave at six.

When I tell you that Anna was another angel sent to us directly from God, I am not exaggerating. She instantly fell in love with my father and took very good care of him. She stayed awake most nights because he still was not sleeping well. He would get up several times during the night needing to go to the bathroom or just for a drink of water. As he became feebler, less cognitively with it and more scared of dying, Anna sat up holding his hand and comforting him.

So, the bottom line is that I suggest that you not get wrapped up in the "professionalism" of home care companies. For Gene and me, and my father, it was more important to have the right person in our home than it was to have someone who was certified in wiping my father's butt. I would also recommend that you use a friend of a friend. There are many folks looking for work who are willing to help, and unless there is some serious medical care needed, a layperson can be just as effective for much less money.

Chapter Twelve

A Second Ending

Anna and I would sit up and talk when I got home at one o'clock in the morning. I wasn't usually tired right away, so she shared her life with me, and I with her. We became fast friends. She had two sons, and by the glow on her face when she talked about them, I knew she loved them dearly. I loved listening to her talk. She had a thick Polish accent that was intoxicating. Her English was perfect; it just had a Polish lilt.

Every morning she would report to Gene how the night went. In the beginning it was hard because he wasn't sleeping, but the doctor prescribed a sedative to allow him to relax so he could sleep. By the time it started working, he had another episode.

Gene told Anna that if she ever needed him during the night to call his cell phone, which he was now keeping on the bedside table. There were a couple of times she called when my father was asking for Gene. He was usually able to calm Dad down quickly, and he would fall back to sleep. However, one night she called, and he couldn't calm my father down. He was having a hard time breathing and was in duress. I had only been in bed for a couple of hours, so I stayed upstairs while Gene went down to look in on my dad. He came up a short time later and said he was taking my father to the hospital. He was having a hard time breathing and having stomach pains. He brought my cell phone up so he could call me with updates.

I woke, startled that my phone was ringing, but it wasn't Gene; it was the hospital calling to get my permission to examine my father. Even though Gene and I were married, I was my father's POA and they said only I could give consent. I said yes and hung up the phone.

I slept for a few hours and woke the next morning to a stream of text messages from Gene. The doctor was concerned because my father's bladder was full, but he wasn't urinating, so they decided to put in a catheter. When they did, what seemed like a quart of urine came out. They weren't sure if there was a blockage or if his prostrate was enlarged and would not allow him to urinate properly. All the same, he did have relief with the catheter.

Again, after discussions with his doctor, it was evident that he was failing quickly. Any kind of intervention would have killed him, so they weren't sure what to do. That is when his doctor put in the orders for hospice care and they moved him to the hospice floor—the same one my mother had been on almost a year earlier. I again breathed a sigh of relief. This was familiar territory. I knew he would be in good hands.

I opened the store the next day, meaning I had to be at work at 4:30 in the morning. At around 6:30, I texted my boss—he was an early riser—and told him what was happening.

"My father is on the hospice floor and I'll need to go sign paperwork." He told me to do what I needed.

I left work at around 8:30, once I got things opened and running smoothly. My drive to the hospital seemed to take forever, but I took advantage of the time to get my head together. I was facing my second parent in hospice care in less than a year. By the time I arrived, I had my head wrapped around the idea.

A Second Ending

When my mother died, I told Gene that I didn't think my father would last a year. He said I was crazy; he thought my father would be around for at least another five years. At the time, I hoped he was right, but the recent turn of events made that seem very unlikely.

When I entered his room, Dad was resting comfortably. His room was large and inviting. Soft music was playing in the background, and the smell of brownies was in the air. I swore they were piping the smell through the duct system. Diana, his nurse, came in shortly after I arrived. She updated me on what was going on.

My father had congestive heart failure, so they were giving him Lasix to reduce the fluid around his heart. Since fluid around the heart can cause pain, administering the drug was certainly within the realm of palliative care. She said he was responding well, beginning to eat, but still very confused. She explained that some of the confusion may be caused by the lower sodium levels. It was something we saw from time to time, and she assured me it would get better with time, but I wasn't sure how much time we had.

I left Gene visiting with my father, while Diana and I went to the family room to fill out paperwork. I was very familiar with the process, after having done it for my mother, so we breezed through it. She explained that while my father was under medical care he could stay on the floor, but as soon as no medical intervention was needed, he would have to be released. This meant Gene and I would have to prepare for his release.

For some reason, my father's illness scared me more than my mother's had. Perhaps it was because it had been such a short time since my mother had died; we hadn't caught our breath. For a hot second, I considered putting my father back into the rehab center, but I knew he would be miserable and that would have been a hell of a way to die.

So, we prepared to bring him to our home again. The only thing we needed was a hospital bed. We already had everything else or had it on order. The hospital had him transported by ambulance, and the EMTs helped get him into bed. He rested there for the remainder of the day. Gene helped him eat a couple of times, but he slept most of the day.

We had Anna come to spend the night with him. Although he no longer had to go to the bathroom because of the catheter, my father kept her busy. He wasn't sleeping much at all. He was vocal about not wanting to sleep for fear that he wouldn't wake up. Gene consulted with the hospice nurse, who recommended we start my father on Lorazepam, a drug used to ease anxiety. They also prescribed morphine for any pain he might be in.

By this time, they had stopped all the other medication he was on. The premise was that those meds were designed to keep people alive. Even though my father wasn't actively dying, his time was limited. His heart was failing, and it was only a matter of time before one of the heart attacks would end his life. It felt like we were living with a ticking time bomb.

Things took a turn for the worse on a Wednesday night. My father was uncomfortable and unable to sleep. Gene called hospice, and they suggested we up his dose of morphine and Lorazepam. Once we did, he settled down.

The next morning, his nurse came to check on him. Gene and I decided that the night before was very difficult on my father, that the current routine of reacting to his pain was not working. It caused him too much anxiety. I proposed the idea of being proactive, suggesting we give him Lorazepam on a consistent basis to stabilize his anxiety. She agreed, and we mapped out a plan. She said she would be back in the morning to assess his new baseline. He slept most of the day and only ate once. He took sips of water only a couple times that day.

A Second Ending

On Friday, I had a meeting to attend. I needed to leave early in the morning, before the nurse arrived. When she did arrive, she let Gene know that my father was actively dying. This was their way of letting the family know that death was only hours away. We'd heard the same term when my mother was in her final hours. After looking in on him before I left, I wasn't convinced he would still be alive when I returned home after my meeting.

I got home around three o'clock that afternoon. I went in to check on him immediately. His breathing was slow but consistent. The nurse had told Gene to start giving him morphine every four hours. Since his breathing was labored and his lungs were crackling, the nurse wanted to make sure he was comfortable.

Saturday morning came. Gene and I both woke up early. Here's where I'll make my confession. During both my parents' illnesses, Gene was the strength in our partnership. He never wavered from his duties as caregiver, although he complained from time to time. but who wouldn't; he was stuck in the house with my father, who wasn't making sense most of the time, and try as he may, he was never able to ease my father's fear of dying. So, when we woke, I waited in the living room while he went to check on my father. He was still alive. He was only breathing two or three times a minute, but he was still breathing. We settled in for what would be a very long day.

When he wasn't taking care of my parents, Gene is a sports broadcaster. He is superb at his job and has been called an artist at his trade by many fans he has met. On that Saturday, he had a game around four o'clock. He considered cancelling, but I insisted he go.

"Look, he's going to die when he's damn good and ready. It won't matter if you're here or not, so go. It'll do you good to get out of the house," I insisted.

He had been giving my father morphine every four hours as instructed by the nurse. She had stopped by earlier in the day and helped Gene turn my dad so that the gurgling stopped.

For Christmas, Gene had bought me a video game for our PS4 that I wanted. It was a farming game where you plow fields, sow seeds, and harvest crops for money. For most who dabble in the video game world, it would have been sheer boredom, but for me, it was a make-believe world I could control and a way to pass the hours on my day off.

That Saturday, it was what got me through. Every fifteen minutes or so I would check on my father. From the threshold of his bedroom door, I waited to see if his chest was moving. All day it was the same, two or three breaths every minute. I noticed his forehead was crinkled; he was fighting.

When my mother died, I knew she wanted to be alone. I sensed that the last time I looked in on her. It's how most people go, by themselves. I think it's so their loved ones don't experience their last breath.

At eight o'clock that night when Gene got home from work, my father was still alive. I'm not sure why it dawned on me when it did, but I realized that my father was not going to die if he was alone. He was afraid of dying; he'd made that very clear.

"He's not going to go unless I am in there with him," I said to Gene.

I poured myself a glass of wine and went to his room. His breathing was down to two breaths every minute. I found myself holding my breath between his breaths. I sat down in the pink chair next to his bed and took his hand. It was warm, warmer than his hand had been in years. I assumed it was from some fever that was running through his body. Nonetheless, it felt good compared to my mother's cold hand when she was at this stage.

A Second Ending

I sat there holding his hand and speaking to him through my thoughts. I told him he needed to let go, that I was going to be okay and it was his time to go. I told him he could stop worrying and that there was nothing to be afraid of. I asked him to say hello to everyone who went to heaven before him and told him he would have a great time reconnecting with loved ones.

It was only thirty minutes or so after I sat next to him that I watched my father take his last breath. It was nothing like I had imagined. For some reason, I thought dying would be much more dramatic than it was. Perhaps that was from only seeing it happen on TV. In fact, after taking his last breath, his crinkled forehead smoothed out; he looked so peaceful. I looked at the clock; it was 9:09 p.m. on September 9. I smiled. To me, this was a sign that his transition was complete and he was in heaven where he deserved to be.

I kissed him on the forehead and went out to the living room. "He's gone," I said quietly to Gene.

"What? You just went in there," he exclaimed.

"I knew he was waiting for me to be with him," I said with tears in my eyes. We hugged for a few minutes. It was finally over.

While I never envisioned my parents dying in my home when I decided to move back to care for them, it happened that way. With Gene's help and constant support and encouragement, I could fulfill both my parents' wishes to die at home peacefully, surrounded by love.

I picked up my cell phone and dialed the number for hospice.

Chapter Thirteen

Funeral Preparations

When we started this journey, Gene and I discovered that my parents hadn't made any arrangements for their deaths. It was as if they thought if they didn't prepare, it wouldn't happen. In June, we took matters into our own hands. Gene found out that there were still a couple of plots left in the small Laysville Cemetery located at the beginning of the street where they had lived together for the last fifty-four years. While we never discussed it, I felt it was only appropriate that they be buried there.

My mother was not a religious person. She believed in God but had stopped practicing any religion years earlier. After I was born, she went on birth control pills. Back then, the Catholic Church frowned upon anyone using birth control of any kind. The church believed it was messing with God's plan. My mother thought differently.

Living in a small town was great from many perspectives, but when it got back to the priest of the church we attended, it wasn't so great. The first time my mother was refused communion during a church service was the last time she set foot in a church. She felt that her religion had judged her and turned its back on her, so she did the same.

When it came to planning for my mother's funeral, I took all of this into consideration. She would not have wanted a Catholic

Funeral Preparation

mass, even though my father wanted that for her, so we settled for a graveside service said by a Catholic priest.

It was a chilly morning in December. My aunt had arranged for a priest from her church to come to the cemetery. We only invited Gene's mother and my aunt. It's what my mother would have wanted. She never wanted anyone to make a fuss over her.

Some may think it ironic, but I did not, that the priest who came was an older Irish gentleman. As we gathered around the gravesite, I laid my mother's ashes on the ground and sprayed yellow roses around her biodegradable urn. Yellow was her favorite color.

If you've never had to make choices about how to dispose of someone's remains, there are far more options than I had imagined. Two days after she died, I met with the undertaker to look at options for her burial. Since there would be no wake and no church service, I thought it would be simple, but there were still a lot of choices I needed to make—and fees associated with each of those choices, of course.

I won't go into everything here, but I will tell you that the one choice I found interesting was how I wanted my mother's body transported from the funeral home to the crematory. I could choose anything from a cardboard box straight up to a very expensive casket. The undertaker explained that no matter which I chose, it would be burned with my mother's ashes, so I chose a simple pine box. She would not have wanted me to spend tons of money just to have it go up in flames.

I also had to choose what type of urn my mother's ashes would be put into. Again, the choices ranged from a brown cardboard box to a marble urn that cost thousands of dollars. The option that intrigued me was the biodegradable urn. It was a large envelope that was made of something like papier-mâché, with a bag inside made of the same material as a Tylenol capsule. The premise was that once the first rain came, the envelope and the capsule would disintegrate, and her ashes would return to the earth.

I was instantly reminded that the Bible clearly states in Genesis 3:19: "In the sweat of thy face shalt thou eat bread, till thou return unto the ground; for out of it hast thou taken: for dust thou art, and unto dust shalt thou return." It seemed like the perfect choice.

Father Mike started the service with an old Irish hymn. I found it interesting that even though he didn't know my mother, who was one-hundred-percent Irish, he started her service in the most appropriate way he could have. I knew she was smiling.

It was the first time since she died that my father and I cried. While we both knew she was gone, this made it final. I held on to him tightly as Father Mike recited the Catholic graveside service. At the end, we all sang "Amazing Grace." The service was simple and poignant, just as she would have wanted.

After the service was over, we all went to The Shack, a small family-owned joint on the Connecticut shoreline with a great breakfast menu. We went there many times with my parents; it was a favorite spot. It was late morning, so having breakfast in her memory seemed only appropriate.

Once the waitress brought our coffee, we all raised our cups. "To Toots," I said, choking back the tears.

We ate breakfast and chatted. I felt her presence and found great comfort in knowing she was there watching over us as we began the next chapter, this one without her.

***

My father never talked about what he wanted, but I knew he wanted a more traditional burial. He wanted to be buried in a coffin and have a service involving a Catholic priest.

Funeral Preparation

My father's side of the family used the same funeral home for years. I figured all the years of my family investing in outlandish, open-casket, embalmed body, full-Catholic-mass funerals would afford me a family discount. Similar to when my mother died, employees from the funeral home came and picked up my father's body when he died. I went and met with the undertaker after church. Gene went with me. Instead of the cremation process, I had to decide where my father's body would lie for eternity. I chose a modest casket for my father's body, no calling hours, a graveside service, the simplest of burials, and I wrote a check for eight thousand five hundred dollars.

Then there's the headstone. We chose a simple stone shared by my mother and father. It cost over twenty-five hundred dollars. Do some quick math: to bury both my parents, it cost over ten thousand dollars. That's not a sum of money most folks have lying around. If you're lucky enough to have life insurance to cover costs, consider yourself blessed. In my parent's case, their life insurance totaled four thousand dollars. Yes, you're right, the other six thousand came right out of pocket.

Chapter Fourteen

The Practical Piece

Caring for sick parents, or any person for that matter, is not for the faint of heart. It requires a strong reserve, accepting that there is nothing glamorous about it, and that there will be times when you want to throw in to towel for no other reason than it's downright hard.

There are some practical things that you'll need to know to make the journey easier. Hopefully, this chapter will provide some practical advice on what you'll need.

Insurance

Medical insurance is also something you'll want to look at early on. Hopefully, insurance is in place that will cover bills. My parents had Medicare and supplemental insurance that covered what Medicare didn't, which helped, but it didn't cover everything. Medical bills add up quickly. Remember that ten-day stint that my mother had in the hospital where literally nothing happened? That bill was well over seventy thousand dollars. Most people don't have that kind of nest egg laying around, neither did my parents. Luckily my mother made sure they had the supplemental, so that their responsibility was just a few thousand—but it was still a few *thousand*.

Two Sets of Bills

It was during a visit to my parents' home in February 2016 that I realized that my mother had all but stopped taking care of their finances. Mail was piling up near the chair where she sat. When I started going through it, all the bills had unpaid balances in addition to the current bill. My mother had always been a stickler for paying things on time. She had a system that tracked their expenses that she had used for years. She kept every bill, cancelled check, and bank statement neatly filed in the desk in her office. I was quite alarmed when I realized that most of their bills were past due.

I knew that I would have to take over for her, since my father had never paid a bill in his life. His parents did it when he was young, and my mother assumed that duty when they married. I quickly took matters into my own hands and started sorting the pile of mail that had accumulated. I found it funny that my parents received tons of requests for donations to various charities. I'm not quite sure if they donated to all of them, but I know my mother was quite conservative with their meager retirement. After everything was sorted, I sat down with my mother's checkbook and paid all the past due bills. My father sat with me at the dining room table and signed all the checks.

It took me a couple of months to get their bills straightened out. As I said, most of them were past due by the time I got involved, but I corrected it quickly and got into the rhythm of paying their bills on time. Once they both moved in with us, I had their mail forwarded to my home and even changed the billing address on most of their accounts. It just made life easier.

I'll interject here that you'll want to get usernames and passwords for things like email addresses or other accounts they may have online. While there weren't many for my parents, with their simple way of living, online accounts could add up quickly if your parents are more involved in using the computer. If you have a POA, you have the legal right to access any accounts online, so get the passwords.

In my mother's case, she had a few bills that were sent to her by email. While there were only a couple, they were very important, like the insurance on their car and home, or the monthly statement from their oil company. Having her username and password for her email account made it easy for me to check it periodically to make sure nothing got missed.

Power of Attorney

It was shortly after this that I knew I would oversee my parents' finances. I consulted with my attorney, who suggested that my parents appoint me as their power of attorney. Since I was not only taking care of their bills but also helping my mother make medical decisions, he felt I needed legal authority to ask questions and get answers to questions that may be protected by HIPAA laws.

There are different types of power of attorney documents. The POA can be restricted to only financial decisions or only medical decisions. In my parents' case, they opted to give me full power to make any decisions they were not able to make for themselves. I am happy to report that neither of my parents ever got to a point where they couldn't make decisions on their own. This made my job much easier, because I only had to make sure that their wishes came to fruition.

POA documents must always be kept up to date. Most banking institutions and hospitals will only honor a POA if it has been executed within a year. After that, they will look for it to be updated, even if there is no end date noted within the document.

The Practical Piece

After my mother died, I legally changed my name back to my maiden name, so my father had to execute another POA with my new legal name. Then I had to file the new document with his bank.

I got in the habit of carrying a copy of the POA with me. There were several times throughout the year that I was glad I had it on me.

It's important to note that a POA document is only valid while the person is alive. At the time of death, it is no longer valid, making you powerless to make decisions. You may want to consider being added as a joint owner on any account. This allows you to have access to funds after death, without having to go through probate. In my father's case, it allowed me to have funds to pay for his funeral without having to involve probate.

My parents had never jumped on the Internet train. They still had dial-up Internet service, and even though my mother had a debit card, she admitted that she'd never used it. She paid everything by check or cash, only using charge cards to delay payments on large purchases. They clearly never got the "American Dream" memo about living beyond their means, swiping a card to pay for everything and paying their bills electronically.

I, on the other hand, apart from living beyond my means, was all about the convenience of debit cards and online bill paying. It only took me thirty days to get them up to speed. Having the ability to pay their bills from my computer, rather than sit and write checks, may sound minor, but it allowed me to spend the limited time I had during visits to make sure their house was clean and that they had what they needed to make it a few days until my next day off.

It's important to get a feel for what the monthly expenses are, the income to cover them, and if there is a shortage. It's also equally as important to know what kind of income is coming in, whether it be Social Security, pensions, or the like. In my parents' case, they had adequate money to cover their expenses, at least when they were healthy. The good news is that they had a little nest egg set aside to cover any unforeseen bills that would arise from illness or the upkeep of their home.

Where are the Important Documents?

I'll admit I was cautious about asking my parents about their finances. I didn't want them to think I was prying into their personal information. They were extremely open and trusting with me. They knew I only had their best interests in mind. It's important to have that kind of relationship when you're taking charge of someone's finances and medical decisions.

It's equally as important to know where important documents are kept. My mother, being the organized person she was during most of her years, kept all their important papers in a locked box that she stored in the back of her closet behind an old shoe box. It contained every legal document they had ever signed, their birth certificates, our vaccination charts, my father's military discharge papers (which would come in handy after his death to get a military placard on his grave), their marriage license. You name it, it was in that small locked box.

Find out early where these documents are. You'll need them at some point in your journey, and getting your hands on them while everyone is still functioning cognitively will make your life easier. Then, put them in a safe place. Don't leave them behind for someone else to find.

I also started a file of my own early on. It contained documents like my POA for both my parents, my mother's living will, and a multitude of documents that had to do with legal transactions.

Everything was in one place. It made my life handling not only my own bills, but theirs, much easier. Organization is key.

Medical Equipment

When my mother came to our home in August, we had nothing that would help us; we had to start from scratch. On hospice care, some of what you'll need is covered by insurance. Without sounding too cynical, I assumed they covered a lot, knowing the person would not need coverage for long, and because it's less expensive than being in a skilled nursing facility.

We had them bring in a hospital bed for both my parents. It was just easier and more comfortable than a traditional bed. You'll recall my father was living with us and sharing a room with my mother, so we bought a twin bed that would fit in the room with the hospital bed. For my mother, hospice ordered a wheelchair, which was intricate in her being able to spend time with us in the living room while she was still able.

Both my parents were incontinent during the last months of their life. This is where the glamour ends and the mess begins. Whether it happens at the beginning of a loved one's illness or at the end, it's bound to happen. We experimented with every adult diaper known to man. We found that the underwear type worked best for us. The traditional diaper type was too loose, which allowed things to flow out uncontrollably, if you know what I mean. The underwear type contained whatever was lurking within.

You'll also want to pack in tons of wipes. Don't go the unscented route, you'll want all the perfume you can get to clear the air. Adult urine and feces smell bad. We also found that cutting the sides of the diaper was a better way to get the diaper off, especially when they contained poop. It may sound odd, but we tried it other ways and paid the price by having to clean up more than we needed to. We learned quickly.

Hospital beds don't come with sheets, and regular twin sheets don't fit. You need to buy three sets of hospital sheets. One for the bed, one for the wash, and one just in case. They aren't cheap, so do your research. We bought one set at a local medical supply store; the other two we bought online through Amazon. Once we knew what we needed, we bought most of our supplies that way. You can save a lot of money.

The next thing you'll want to buy is what the nurses in the hospital call chucks. These are quilted rectangles that hospitals put under patients so they can move them up in a bed. With a person on each side of the bed, you can lift a patient by picking up the chuck underneath and sliding them up. It saves backs and makes the process easier on everyone. When it was time to move my mom, we had her fold her arms over her chest; this helped too.

You'll also want to consider buying some disposable bed protection. We did, and it cut down on the laundry and made it easier to clean up.

Be prepared! You'll be doing laundry every day. After sleeping for eight hours, my mother's bed would often smell and be stained with urine. As part of our daily routine, while Gene tended to her morning coffee, I would open the windows and change her bed.

We also bought a buzzer for my mother. Like a nurse's call button, this allowed her to call us in the other room if she needed anything. At first, she thought it funny to push the buzzer for no reason at all. Gene or I would respond and she would giggle, but in all honesty, it gave us peace of mind that if she needed us during the night, we were a buzzer away.

If you have a first-floor bedroom, that is the best option. It may mean moving out if that room happens to be yours, but it will avoid having a hospital bed in the middle of the house. Also, a TV, even if it's a small one, will help your patient pass the time and stop them from constantly pondering their illness.

For years, I tried to get my parents to eat healthier. When they got sick, this was no longer important. What was important for my mother was to find food she would eat that would go down. During the last month of her life, she ate mostly pudding and protein drinks. Be prepared to bring in all the favorites. Fats, nutrition, and carbohydrates no longer matter. What matters is pumping enough calories in to keep the body alive.

The body can go for a period without food, depending on the person's weight, before they became sick, but the human body cannot survive more than three or four days without water. It's important that your patient get as much water as possible. We always had a bottle of water by my mother's bedside table. We offered it to her each time we went in to check on her. Small bottles worked best. It allowed us to monitor her liquid intake and keep it fresh for her. With both my parents, a straw made it easier for them to drink.

Be prepared for change. The needs of both my parents changed often while they were sick. As time went on, they required more assistance from Gene and I to care for them. Be adaptable; you'll need it.

If your insurance covers it, do not hesitate to accept help from professional healthcare services like visiting nurses and home health aides; they are invaluable. I know that washing up a loved one may seem like a simple task, one that you can handle, but it's also something that you can get help with, which frees you up to do other things, even run a quick errand if needed.

The HHAs are scheduled through the local visiting nurse association, after the initial intake and evaluation. For my mother, we had them come in three times a week. They would give her a sponge bath, wash her hair, put lotion on her (sick people's skin gets dehydrated quickly), change her bed if needed, and just sit with her if Gene needed to run to the store. They were truly an integral part of our success.

Towards the end, we stopped the home health aides for both my parents. When the person moves to the actively dying stage, it's no longer necessary. But on the off chance that you forget to stop the service, they will do just about anything: laundry, light housework, just sitting with the patient, etc.

As you can imagine, having both parents living with us, me still working sixty hours a week, and Gene doing most of the caregiving, left little time for much else. That included general housework in a household with four adults and three cats. We bit the bullet and hired a housekeeper. You can find one that will come in once a month for about $125, and it will be well worth it. While Gene and I couldn't afford the added expense, my parents could, so it was their contribution to our monthly expenses.

I'm sure there will be other things you'll find in your journey that will make this process easier, but these suggestions will set you in the right direction.

The Will and Probate

Along with the emotions that come when a loved one dies, there are a lot of details that need to be taken care of. My parents died within ten months of each other, so my mother's estate was not even completed when my father died.

My mother had a will and left everything to my father, but there were tasks I needed to complete to file her estate in probate court. For instance, I needed an appraisal on their home in Old Lyme, so the value could be noted on the documents needed.

Even though it was nowhere near the two-million-dollar limit for taxation on an estate, the court still wants an accounting of all assets.

Most of what my mother and father owned was in my father's name, though on some they were listed jointly. This made the probate filing rather easy, with one exception. The caveat to closing my mother's estate stemmed on a small piece of land, a right-of-way for lake access that they had purchased with their neighbors forty years earlier.

When the deed was written, there was no mention of the deed going to my father once my mother died. There was no mention of survivorship. Even though everything went to my father in her will, I was forced to open a full estate so that her ownership of the property could move to my father legally. Her portion of the value was less than two thousand dollars. If I had known, it could have easily been taken care of before she died.

After my mother died, I attempted to file everything in probate myself. As soon as things got a little complicated, (i.e. the small piece of land mentioned earlier), I stepped back and decided I needed to leave this process to the professionals. There are a lot of papers to file, sign, and deliver, most of which the layperson knows nothing about. There are plenty of attorneys that deal with family law who can help, and they are well worth the cost.

Chapter Fifteen

The Spiritual Piece (or Peace)

One of the best things Gene and I had in our toolbox was our strong faith in God. At times, this was the only thing that got us through whatever was happening—like the strokes my mother had in our living room while I was alone with her. It was only the knowledge that God would get us through that episode that kept me from falling apart as it was happening.

I have believed for years that everything happens for a reason, that nothing is a coincidence. This is so much of who I am, that I have been writing about my experiences for a couple of years. In my blog, *His Mysterious Ways*, I recount many things that have happened over the years that have not been a coincidence. Whether it's people I meet or circumstance that happen, it is for a greater purpose.

I've found throughout my life that things that happen to me, good or bad, are meant to give me knowledge that will allow me to help someone later in my life. I look for the lesson in the trials and joys that come my way. For instance, the time my oldest son developed a gangrenous appendix. The six weeks of wandering through the medical system, and dealing with weeks of his healing, helped me later in life when a friend's daughter got ill and when my parents got sick.

I think it's important to have a spiritual outlook when going through something like taking care of a sick loved one. Knowing

The Spiritual Piece (or Peace)

that there is a higher power can keep you grounded and purposeful during what can be an extremely hard time. However, it's important to keep in mind that we all have different spiritual needs.

For all his life, my father continued to attend Sunday mass at the Catholic church in town. He liked the ritual nature of the religion; it gave him comfort. But I never got the sense that he had a close relationship with God. When we talked about his fear of dying, he never found comfort in God's plan or that he would eventually end up in heaven.

During his illness, his comfort came when a priest visited him, or a layperson brought him communion. I found it interesting that when I suggested that he pray about something, he would recite the Lord's Prayer or a round of Hail Marys. He did his fair share of "Please, God, help me" also, but I don't think he ever knew what he was asking for. I'm not sure if he wanted God to help him live or help him die.

My father met with a spiritual leader in our home during what would be the last week of his life. I was at work, but Gene was there and filled me in on the meeting. She asked him if he felt he needed to ask for forgiveness for anything. He was very emphatic, saying he didn't need forgiveness, and he was right. My father led the life of a man committed to his family, devoted to my mother, even if she didn't deserve it at times. He was a hard worker and honored God in his own way.

When the spiritual leader asked him if there was anyone he needed to forgive, he pondered the question for a moment. "I guess I need to forgive my other children," he said. They talked about what happened with my brother and sister, and then he prayed that God would stay close to them and help them through their own specific journeys.

I talked to my dad about the experience. He was fuzzy on the details but did remember that they spoke about my brother and sister. I thought this might bring up his need to see them, but it didn't. It was as if he had forgiven them for the years of pain they caused, and he was at peace.

My mother, on the other hand, had given up on religion years ago. Her relationship with God was much more personal. During the last weeks of her life, I asked her if she was talking to God. She told me she was, and when I asked her what she was talking about, she told me that was between her and God. I often wondered if she was spending her time asking for forgiveness—not that I think she needed any special dispensation for the life she led. Just like my father, she stood by him in sickness and in health. She raised us the best way she knew how, she was a good friend, and in her own way, she was very giving.

For me, my unyielding faith in God, the knowledge that he only gives you what you can handle, and that he is there for you each step of the way, are the most important parts of my spiritual being. Believing that he had my journey planned out before I took my first breath allows me to take my hands off the wheel and let him drive.

In the early stage of my journey with my parents, there were times when my little Anglican church in the schoolhouse gym was the only place I felt safe. During one service, after receiving communion, I broke down. Father Jay has an uncanny way of knowing when I need extra prayers. I'm not quite sure if his sense came from just knowing or if someone was filling him in, but he always knew when I needed assurance that I was on the right path.

It's important to also appreciate and celebrate the faith that your patient practices. For both my parents, this looked different, but I could respect each of their unique spiritual needs and instill some of my beliefs to give them comfort.

For me, God's love constantly surrounded my family as he walked us through some of the most difficult times in our lives.

The Spiritual Piece (or Peace)

He allowed me the opportunity to serve my parents in a way I had never imagined, during some of the humbling times of their lives. It was then that I finally understood what he meant by "honor thy mother and thy father."

When he came up with this commandment, there were no stipulations or clauses in that phrase. In other words, he didn't say "honor thy mother and father only if they are the people you want them to be." I finally understood that my parents did the best they could during my upbringing, that I am the person I am today because of their commitment to raising me, and that I had an opportunity to pay it forward by caring for them.

I truly consider this time as a gift. It gave me an opportunity to see my parents at their most vulnerable state, when they were dying. It gave me an opportunity to learn more patience (although my husband may disagree), trust, and faith in our most merciful God.

The religion doesn't matter. What matters is your faith that God is there for you as you go through this time and that he will be with those you love forever, even after they die.

Chapter Sixteen

The Relationship Effect

If you're lucky enough to have a partner to help you with the daily tasks of helping a sick parent, consider it a blessing. When I say I never would have been able to take care of my parents without Gene, it's an understatement. Working sixty hours a week and taking care of a sick person doesn't exactly work. If he hadn't been semi-retired with a job that allowed him to work from home, my parents would have been forced to live out the last year of their lives in a nursing home.

With all the gratefulness that I feel for having Gene along on this journey with me, there were times when it was extremely difficult. Both he and I are extremely opinionated, so if we disagreed about something that was going on, there was usually a heated discussion about the subject.

Then there were all the emotions I personally felt. There was guilt because Gene was bearing the brunt of our decision. He was the one doing the daily care, taking care of their needs, feeding them, laundry, grocery shopping, etc. I got up each morning and made sure my mother was cleaned up from the night before, but that was the extent of my responsibilities. I went to work each day and left him behind to care for my parents.

When I said in the Preface that caring for a sick parent isn't for the faint of heart, I meant it. There aren't many people I know who would be willing to take on the task of caring for someone else's parents, which included personal care, cooking two or three different meals a day, and having to yell all the time for two people who had hearing problems; you get the picture.

I can tell you that the keys to making sure your relationship makes it through the journey are lots of patience, open communication, and a lot of understanding. Also, there needs to be an understanding that any situation is not about you; it's about the person you're caring for.

Chapter Seventeen

Pay it Forward

Everything happens for a reason, and everything happens at the right time. Life isn't what we expect it to be, or even how we perceive it in our minds. For instance, if you envision something, it may come to you in a slightly different way. I'll give you an example.

After my divorce, I asked God to bring someone into my life that I could share it with. I wanted someone who loved family, was smart and funny. If anyone told me those traits would come to me in Gene's body, someone I'd known thirty years earlier, I would have told them they were high. But that's how it happened, and I thank God every day.

When things happen in my life that I know have an underlying lesson, I store that information for use later in life. I know others do too.

Like my friend Celenia, who I work with. You see, she walked the same path as me earlier in life when she took care of her mother. Celenia is a Puerto Rican woman whose smile lights up the room, and her positive attitude is infectious. She lives life through rose-colored glasses. Her glass is always half full, and she's never had a bad day. We're like soul sisters.

When I started this journey with my mother, Celenia was a great resource for me. After all, she had already been through it. She knew the system, how to navigate it, and empathized with my frustration. She also knew the emotional end of it. She was patient as I bawled my way through this phase or that phase. It was a true blessing that she showed up in my life at the perfect time. I'll be eternally grateful.

Chapter Eighteen

Closure

Each time something tragic happens in someone's life, there has to be closure. Whether it's a divorce, an accident, or the death of a loved one, it is a healing time that lets a person move on from sadness back into the light. Everyone perceives closure differently. It's a very personal thing.

As you read in my earlier chapter, I experienced a lot of frustration and anger when I was navigating the medical system. I have yet to understand how a system that holds people's lives in their hands can be so cold, rigid, and arrogant. From my mother's primary care physician, to hospital staff, to specialists, there were very few people I encountered who truly cared about my mother's health. The robotic nature of the medical system is a cold, uncaring place, except for hospice.

Shortly after my mother died, I got a call from her doctor's management group. A woman named Susan called, concerned that my parents had left the care of their doctor.

As my parents' POA, I had made the decision to find a new doctor for them. The decision was made because so many things were screwed up during my mother's illness, and many of these screwups were a direct result of their doctor's unwillingness to speak to me directly. When I received Susan's call, I knew it was an opportunity for me to have someone hear my story. During our thirty-minute conversation, I relayed the chain of events that led up to my decision to remove my parents from her managed account to someone who might care.

At the end of the conversation, I was hopeful that something good would come out of all my distress. Susan assured me she would open a case, look into things, and get back with me. She even sent me an email expressing her concerns and confirming that she would follow up. I was hopeful.

> *Barb,*
>
> *Thank you again for taking the time to speak with me today.*
>
> *I am very sorry for your loss and for the additional stress related to your Mom's healthcare journey.*
>
> *As we discussed, I will begin to do a complete quality of care review and will then follow up with you.*
>
> *We will use your feedback to provide education on the importance of making a human connection and being caring and compassionate in every interaction.*
>
> *This process generally takes 2-3 weeks. If it looks like it is going to take longer than that, I will send you an interim letter to update you on my progress.*
>
> *Please share your address with me so that I have that if I need it.*
>
> *Thanks again for sharing your Mom's story with me.*
>
> *Take care,*
> *Susan*

Weeks went by before there was any further communication from Susan. Furthermore, the only reason that communication was reopened was because I initiated it. After leaving a voicemail for her and sending a follow up email, she contacted me.

The gist of the conversation was that she had relayed my information to Dr. Smith's superior for review. When I asked what would happen, she was very vague. When I probed further, she let me know that it was unlikely that there would be any disciplinary action, and on the off chance that there was, I would not be privy to that information.

I requested a meeting with Dr. Smith, his superior, and Susan. While Susan said she would relay my request, I knew it was not likely to happen. I never heard from her again.

I tried to let it go. I know that harboring ill feelings towards someone is not healthy. Get mad and get over it. But in this case, I just couldn't come to terms with the thought of this man not knowing how he had affected me and my family. Months later, I took the time to compose a letter. Here is what I said:

May 28, 2017
Dr. Smith
RE: Elizabeth Lorello

Dear Dr. Smith:
Since I was not afforded the opportunity to meet with you directly, I feel compelled to write this letter in an effort to have some closure with the issue of my mother's care under you. I will thank you in advance for taking the time to read this in its entirety.
I'll begin by stating that I understand that my mother may not have been one of your easiest patients. She was very set in her ways and tended to muscle her way through life. That being said, when I read the Hippocratic Oath nowhere did it state that you would only treat cooperative patients. Among other things, you were charged to fulfill by taking that

Closure

oath, it clearly states, "I will remember that I do not treat a fever chart, a cancerous growth, but a sick human being, whose illness may affect the person's family and economic stability. My responsibility includes these related problems, if I am to care adequately for the sick."

In January of 2016, my mother contacted your office regarding the fact that she was vomiting when she ate. She was not granted an appointment with you until a month later. I would have thought that word that one of your patients vomiting on a regular basis would have caused more of a sense of urgency to get her into your office. That being said, from that point you sent her a specialist for an endoscopy, which was inconclusive, although she was diagnosed with achalasia. Her next appointment with you was scheduled in April 2016, four months after her initial call to your office.

On April 6, 2016, I called your office attempting to get an email address for you so I could send you information regarding my mother's condition. I was told that your staff did not give out your email address. When I explained my reason for wanting it, I was again denied. How, in this day and age, can you not have an email address that you are willing to give patients? Please keep in mind that in 2014 both my parents signed consent for you to give me access to their files and to discuss their care with you. I am enclosing a copy of the email I wanted to send you so that you understand what my concerns were early on.

When I told your receptionist that I wished to speak with you before my mother's upcoming appointment, and that I was willing to pay up to $300 for an hour of your time, I was once again denied. I did however receive a call the day before my mother's appointment extending an invitation to come to the appointment, which I had already planned on attending, at my mother's request.

If you will recall that appointment was to discuss the possibility of doing a motility test under sedation, since my mother was opposed to being awake during the procedure. This would have been the final deciding factor for her diagnosis so we could proceed with treatment. The motility test was scheduled for July 18, 2016, even though I continued to stress my concerns about waiting that long.

Between April 6, 2016 and June 29, 2016, I called your office over thirty times, often times asking to speak to you directly regarding my mother's health. Not once did you return my phone call. In fact, to add insult to injury, during that time frame I never was able to speak with you and didn't hear from you until the murmurs of cancer reached you.

During the time we were waiting for the all-conclusive motility test, my mother was losing weight at warp speed. She lost over thirty pounds from her visit with you in February until I admitted her to Hartford Hospital in late June. She was barely keeping food down, often times vomiting even water. In June, I took matters into my own hands and admitted her to Hartford Hospital, where she was diagnosed with malnutrition and dehydration. She spent ten days there while they tried to stabilize her.

Needless to say, the journey my family took during my mother's illness was a roller coaster ride, from your staff getting instructions wrong about specialists, to the rigid way in which this whole thing was handled, to watching my mother wither away. It was a challenging eleven months, during which I never felt I had your support or the support of your staff.

My mother died of gastric cancer on November 12, 2016, eleven months after her initial call to you.

All this being said, you may be wondering why I am taking the time to write this. My hope is that by pointing out

Closure

> these missteps, your future patients, and their families, will not have to go through what my family did. You inherited many geriatric patients when you took over Dr. X's practice. With that, you have also inherited a generation of offspring who are fairly educated (although not as you in the medical profession) and have questions that must be answered when tasked with caring for aging parents.
>
> Thank you for your time.
> Barbara Lorello
> cc: Chairman of the Advisory Board
> Susan / Patient Experience Specialist

About a week after Dr. Smith received my letter, I received a response in the mail. It was short and sweet. He sent his condolences on my loss, apologized for anything that may have made things more difficult for my family, said he was open to a face-to-face discussion, and left it at that.

I never had that face-to-face with him. I didn't feel anything good would come of it. My mother taught me years ago that if you don't have anything nice to say, don't say anything at all. I left it at that.

***

This is the email I referred to in the letter. I never got to send it to him in April when I wrote it:

> Good Morning Dr. Smith:
> My name is Barbara Lorello-Rollar. I am Elizabeth Lorello's youngest (now 53 years old) daughter. As I understand it, you have taken over my mother's health care with the retirement of Dr. X.

Let me begin by letting you know that I completely understand that discussing my mother's health is a violation of HIPAA laws and I would never ask anyone to violate any law. My purpose here is not to discuss my mother's health with you, but to provide you with some information that you may not have. If you already have this information, I apologize for taking your time, but rest assured that my mother's health is of my utmost concern.

As you have probably already surmised by this time, my mother is a hard nut to crack. While I won't go into the history behind her attitude, suffice it to say that we won't teach an old dog (no disrespect meant) new tricks. That being said, I would like to make sure you have all the facts, not just what she wants you to know.

If you've had a chance to read my mother's file, you'll find that Dr. X has been treating her for depression for over twenty years with a cocktail of Prozac and Zanex I believe. My research on these medications indicated that they should be used in conjunction with therapy, but for whatever reason, my mother and Dr. X agreed to bypass that part; most likely because my mother doesn't want to talk about it.... Shocking LOL.

As you know, my mother recently was diagnosed with Achalasia. She told me that you're trying to treat the symptoms of the disorder with a prescription, which you've had some success using with other patients. My research didn't suggest this medication, I read about Viagra and Botox as possibilities for relief. That being said, I am not a doctor, so I trust that you have experience with this medication being used to help with this very rare disorder. (I can't believe there are only 200,000 cases recorded)

On Saturday, April 2, I visited my parents at their home in Old Lyme, approximately one week after she started taking the new medication. I was shocked at my mother's appearance.

Normally my mother looks pale because she rarely goes outside; her depression has gotten worse since she has gotten older. But when I saw her on Saturday, her face was droopy and she looked exhausted. She seemed more lethargic than normal and my father said she was having a hard time getting up off the couch by herself.

My mother had kept the sheet of paper containing the laundry list of side effect of the medication you are trying with her and two of them really stuck out. The first was that the drug caused drowsiness, and the second was that it could cause suicidal tendencies in people prone to suicidal thoughts. I am not sure if you were aware, but my mother was admitted to Middlesex Hospital twenty-five +/- years ago for depression and the fact that she felt suicidal after my father was diagnosed with cancer.

The good news is she thinks the medication may be working. Although I question that since she was vomiting the entire hour of my visit. I am hoping the medication will work and that perhaps it is the type of medication that needs to build up in her system in order to be effective. Since the precautions state she should not just stop taking it, I assume that means it has to build up in her system to be effective.

My first concern is that my mother will not tell you what the side effects are doing to her, especially if she begins to get relief from the vomiting, which is really messing up her quality of life as you can imagine. The second is that this medication will exacerbate her depression, which I believe borders on clinical, manic, or bi-polar on any given day.

My ask is that you keep a very close eye on my mother's medical condition. She can go downhill very quickly and will probably not notify your office until it may be too late. I know her condition is not curable, and I know she is not open to all of the possibilities available to give her a better quality of life.

I also know she is a VERY stubborn old Irish woman. Her relationship with Dr. X was like something from War of the Roses and she liked him because she felt she could tell him what to do. I'm not asking you to foster that same Doctor/Patient relationship with her because quite frankly I think she told me that to make herself feel superior. For whatever that is worth. I often tell her you get more bees with honey than with vinegar, but as I said before, you can't teach an old dog new tricks.

I have asked my mother to contact your office if she doesn't start feeling more energetic in the next week or so. I have also asked my father to keep a close eye on her and call me if she doesn't improve (BTW I live five minutes from Middlesex Hospital in Middletown and am twenty minutes from them). If your practice does wellness calls, please call my mother to see how she is doing. I am sure she will be cranky, and probably caustic, and I will certainly apologize for that in advance.

If she allows me, I will be coming with her for her next visit with you at the end of April. I know she doesn't ask many questions and is easily "disgusted" with the whole process. She isn't a patient patient; I'm sure this is another shocking revelation to you.

I ask that you keep this communication confidential; her paranoia would kick in if she felt you and I were conspiring with each other about her health. I appreciate the time it has taken for you to read this email. I look forward to meeting you in person.

Best regards,
Barbara Lorello-Rollar

Closure

On September 16, 2017, Gene and I went out to dinner alone for the first time in a very long time. It was towards the end of summer in New England, but it was still warm enough for us to enjoy a meal outside at one of our favorite restaurants downtown.

We left our cell phones home. I insisted. I felt we needed to reconnect. The last several years had been centered around my parents and family. While our relationship was still solid, it had been neglected.

That night we spent time chatting about the part of our journey that just ended. Some of the discussion was sad, some poignant, and at other times we laughed. After all, even in the most stressful times, there were still moments of joy and laughter. We agreed on one thing emphatically. We both felt we were blessed to have had the opportunity to care for my parents in our home. There were moments of frustration, but for the most part we took our obligation seriously and lovingly.

People have said that we are saints for what we did for my parents. On the contrary, we are no closer to being saints than the doctors and nurses who helped along the way, or the friends and family who supported us when we needed it. In truth, Gene puts it beautifully: "It's just the right thing to do."

I'll admit there were times when I didn't think I could continue. Watching someone die is not for the faint of heart. It takes strong faith in God and a higher cause. It takes an amazing partner who is willing to help without reservation. And for me, it took me remembering one of the ten rules I live my life by: *Honor thy mother and thy father.*

Review Requested:

If you loved this book, would you please provide a review at Amazon.com and Amazon.co.uk?

CPSIA information can be obtained
at www.ICGtesting.com
Printed in the USA
LVHW091051160220
647092LV00001B/285